D1562457

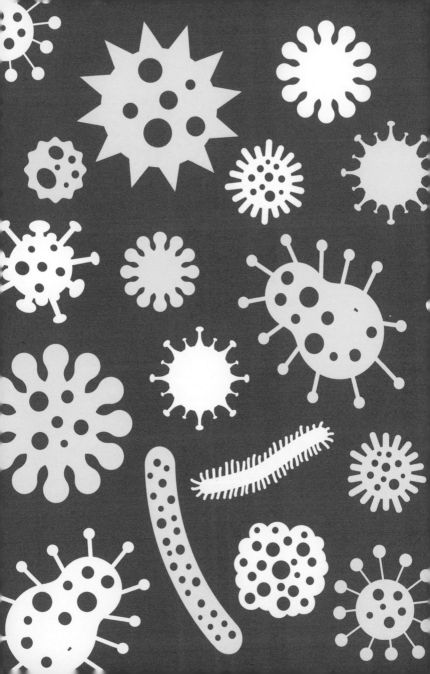

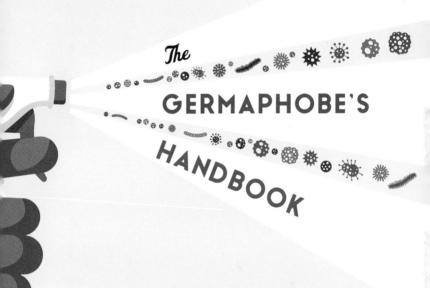

The

GERMAPHOBE'S

HANDBOOK

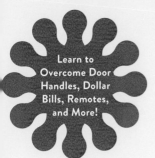

Learn to Overcome Door Handles, Dollar Bills, Remotes, and More!

The

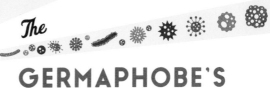

GERMAPHOBE'S

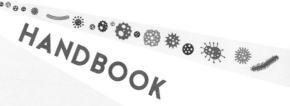

HANDBOOK

AN ENCYCLOPEDIC
SURVIVAL GUIDE
to a
GERM-INFESTED
WORLD

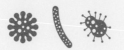

13-digit ISBN: 978-1-95151-118-0
10-digit ISBN: 1-95151-118-2

This book may be ordered by mail from the publisher. Please include $5.99 for postage and handling. Please support your local bookseller first!

Books published by Whalen Book Works are available at special discounts when purchased in bulk. For more information, please email us at info@whalenbookworks.com.

Whalen Book Works
68 North Street
Kennebunkport, ME 04046

www.whalenbookworks.com

Cover and interior design by Melissa Gerber
Typography: Anaheim Gothic, Avenir, Brandon Grotesque, Clarkson Script, Fenway Park and Fontbox Boathouse

Printed in China
1 2 3 4 5 6 7 8 9 0

First Edition

This book is dedicated to anyone who has ever thought twice before touching a public bathroom door.

"Don't let the perfect be the enemy of the good. Lower the bar. Actually spending ten minutes clearing off one shelf is better than fantasizing about spending a weekend cleaning out the basement."

—Gretchen Rubin

TABLE *of* CONTENTS

Chapter 5: Miscellaneous Germs Everywhere 198

INTRODUCTION

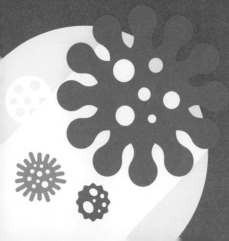

ATTENTION GERMAPHOBES! GERMS ARE EVERYWHERE! THEY'RE HIDING IN PLAIN SIGHT, SITTING ON THE MOST INNOCUOUS OF THINGS, JUST WAITING FOR YOU TO TOUCH THEM AND PICK THEM UP. THEN, THEY WILL HITCH A RIDE WITH YOU, AND DROP OFF ON EVERYTHING YOU TOUCH. THERE'S NO WAY TO ESCAPE THEM . . . HELP!

Well, yes, this is true. Sort of. Viruses are all around and the world is literally swarming with trillions of bacteria. They thrive on just about every surface and even inside of us. In fact, there are more bacteria in our bodies than cells, which brings up the question, what are we, really? But since this isn't a book of philosophy, we'll leave that question to one side, though it may keep you awake at night, more so than worrying about germs! Bacteria are everywhere, but the vast majority of them are neutral to us, or even beneficial. Our bodies couldn't function without all kinds of bacteria in our systems; they literally keep us alive!

We pick up and deposit bacteria all the time, and we come into contact with viruses regularly. In most cases, the bacteria do nothing and our immune systems often knock out viruses so that we never even knew they were there. Regular bacteria are not the problem, it's the pathogens that can do the real damage: E. coli, salmonella, listeria, etc. And in many cases, even these do nothing: we have strains of E. coli in our guts, for example. And our bodies have this wonderful organ called the skin that presents a formidable barrier to anything unpleasant getting in. But nasty things can sometimes get into us, via food, or via our eyes and noses, and when they do, the results can be unpleasant, sometimes deadly. You don't need to consider yourself "germ phobic" to be concerned and want to take actions to protect yourself.

While our modern world has made sanitation a priority, and we generally live in healthier environments than in centuries past, there is no escaping the fact that bacteria, viruses, mold, and other invaders are around us at all times. And this is a good thing, because their presence stimulates our immune systems to respond and keep them out. Many health professionals worry that if someone is brought up in too sterile an environment, they may be less able to fight off infections later on. We evolved to live with these dangers, and our bodies do a good job of keeping us safe most of the time.

That being said, there's no reason why you shouldn't try to keep your home and everything around you as clean as possible. You'll reduce the risk of spreading colds and flu during the season and lower your risk of contracting a dangerous bacterial infection. If you or a loved one is immunocompromised in any way, this can be crucial to maintaining good health. And one of the best ways of keeping your environment cleaner is simply to clean it more often. Yes, that likely made you groan, but it's true!

The good news is that you probably already have a cleaning routine, even if you hate it (you do have a cleaning routine, don't you?). This little book will show you many places in your home and in the world that are potentially unhealthy, and the simple steps you can take to do something about it. Cleaning your home doesn't have to be a massive chore, especially if you do it regularly, and do a little bit every day. And taking a few sensible precautions out in the world will greatly reduce your risk of bringing anything horrible back with you.

Each chapter of this book will give you different places and situations where unwanted visitors could hitch a ride and take up residence in your home or on your possessions. At the end of the book is a glossary of different types of the more dangerous bacteria, as well as a list of the cleaning tools you should have and some of the best cleaners to get the job done.

Due to COVID-19, we've all learned much more about the need for cleanliness, handwashing, etc., as a result of the effects of this virus. That advice holds true at any time. As a result of the pandemic, some of the situations described in this book (staying germ-free in restaurants, bars, and offices) may or may not be relevant to you, but as we move forward, it will be even more necessary to keep those environments clean and to protect ourselves as much as possible. This book is a guide to minimizing risk and ensuring that you and your family are as safe as possible. Let it be your guide to keeping unwanted bacteria and viruses at bay, no matter what kind they are!

CHAPTER 1:

GERMS IN THE HOME

Your home is your castle, but even your castle can't keep out some invaders. Germs and bacteria positively infest everyone's homes. While most of these are harmless, some are pretty unpleasant and hostile, and those are the ones you want to defend your keep against! Whether you live in a studio apartment or a sprawling mansion, developing an effective cleaning routine is essential for keepings things germ-free. In this chapter, we'll look at some of the most common areas in your home that viruses and bacteria can take up residence in, and show you simple ways to ensure that they don't get that toehold. The siege of germs has begun, so here's how to be ready!

YOUR FRONT DOOR

Your door faces the outside world, which means that it can also be a barrier between you and germs, dust, other particles, smoke, and anything else outside. The most obvious way that germs can enter the home is by your door handle. You might not think that the short moments that you open and close your door would matter much, but hidden invaders can be lurking with every touch.

- A single door handle can spread germs to whole buildings in a few hours. Studies of offices have shown that up to 60 percent of people who touched a doorknob and other surfaces picked up the viruses or bacteria on them.

- Another study of commercial door handles found fourteen colonies of bacteria on just one handle, with each colony containing over a million bacteria.

- Studies have shown an alarming increase in the amount of antibiotic-resistant bacteria found on outside door handles.

Obviously, your home isn't likely to have as many visitors and different hands touching the front doorknob, but if you've been out in the world, and opened doors or touched other surfaces, you'll be bringing those germs back with you to your own door handle. Here's what to do.

- Don't touch other things when you come home. Go straight to a sink and wash your hands thoroughly. This will prevent much of whatever you've picked up outside from spreading around.

- Clean your door handle (inside and out) regularly. Use disinfectant wipes with quaternary ammonium compounds (QUATS). These are effective against the flu and other viruses. This is a good idea during flu season and beyond.

- Spray with a disinfectant once a week, and give the handle on both sides a good wipe-down with a cleaning cloth or paper towels.

- These simple steps can reduce the transmission of viruses and bacteria by up to 99 percent! And keeping that many germs out of your home can only be a good thing.

YOUR WELCOME MAT

It may only be the thing you wipe your feet on, but that's the whole problem. When you are out in the world, your shoes pick up and spread a tremendous amount of bacteria and germs, and as you rub the soles of your shoes on your mat, guess what gets transferred to it?

- Studies show that your shoes are far dirtier than you might think. One study showed that in just two weeks, your shoes can acquire over 420,000 units of bacteria! Read more about shoes in chapter 5.

- In that same study, 96 percent of the shoes examined had fecal bacteria. Also found were E. coli and klebsiella pneumoniae, among others.

- Even worse, the transfer rate of those germs and bacteria to your home (especially floor surfaces like tiles) was over 90 percent!

- Other substances, like herbicides and other toxic materials, can also be tracked in.

So, the obvious takeaway is to wipe your feet at the front door, remove your shoes on entering, and have a dedicated place to store them. This should go for you and all visitors to your home. But what about the welcome mat that's getting all of those germs wiped onto it? Obviously, you're going to need to clean it; here's how:

- Be careful not to set other items on it before going into your home, such as grocery bags, handbags, etc. If you must set things down, try to put them on another surface, such as a dedicated chair or box.

Or, if you are not alone, have someone else hold items while you open the door.

- Be sure to wipe your feet on the mat before entering your house. That is what it's there for, after all!

- Shake out your mat regularly. This will dislodge dirt, grass, dust, hair, and anything else you've tracked in or out of the house. Take it away from the house, and, wearing a mask, give it a good beating with a brush to knock out dirt and other particles.

- Sprinkle baking soda onto it, and brush it into the fibers. Let it sit for ten minutes or more, and then shake out the baking soda and give it a thorough brush. This will help eliminate odors and refresh the mat.

- If it's waterproof, rinse it regularly with a hose and let it dry in the sun. Ultraviolet rays are great for killing bacteria.

- Once a week, spray both sides of your mat with a disinfectant to kill germs. Hang it on a clothesline or a similar object, and let it air-dry.

- Be sure to keep the area around the mat clean as well, by sweeping, hosing down, etc.

Done regularly, these simple steps will drastically reduce the amount of germs and bacteria your track into your home.

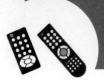

YOUR TV *and* OTHER REMOTE CONTROLS

How many times have you sat on the remote control or lost it in the folds of your crumb-covered couch? Probably too many times to count. Naturally (and grossly!), this leads to a device swarming with invisible germs.

- Studies have shown that the remote may be the dirtiest item in your home!

- That conclusion may seem shocking, but consider: Remotes end up on floors, get sneezed on, get things spilled on them, have pets lick them, get food stuck to them, and any number of other disasters, making them a breeding ground for cold viruses and other infectious nasties. And every time you pick up the remote for any reason, those germs will hop onto your hands.

- This is even truer for remotes in hotels and hospital rooms, where studies suggest that they are actually dirtier than toilets or door handles! Think about all the people who may have used your room's remote before you. Did they all wash their hands properly? Do you have any way to tell? Of course not! And a TV remote is very unlikely to be cleaned properly between occupancies. It's just not something that anyone normally thinks about.

- Just remember that the next time you're staying in a hotel somewhere and want to relax and watch a movie. . . .

Here's what to do to avoid transferring these bugs to your hands:

- Make it a habit to clean the remote, by removing the batteries and wiping the surface down with an alcohol-soaked cotton ball. Let it dry completely before putting back the batteries and using.

- To make cleaning easier, consider purchasing remote covers that can be swapped out every few months. These covers are actually a better option, since remotes—just like computer keyboards—are difficult to clean. Many of these might be washable, or at least you can remove them and clean them with disinfectant.

- Also, try to take better care of your remote to begin with; put it in a dedicated place when you're not using it, watch your food around it, keep out of reach of pets, etc. Yes, this is easier said than done, especially if you have children using it, but taking a bit of extra care at the beginning, when the remote is nice and clean, will prevent the buildup of germs and sticky, yucky messes.

The remote is an essential survival tool these days, so make sure it stays clean. You rely on it so much for your binges, so show it some love, and it'll love you back!

YOUR COMPUTER KEYBOARD

Whether you work on a desktop or a laptop, your fingers will be on your keyboard much of the time. This is true whether you are in an office or are working at home. And like a remote, things get spilled on keyboards, we sneeze and cough in their general direction, and, basically, they can harbor all sorts of stuff from our grubby fingers.

- Research shows that your keyboard, whether desktop or laptop, can be hundreds, if not thousands, of times dirtier than a toilet seat. Ew.

- Even worse, drug-resistant staphylococcus aureus (MRSA) can survive for up to twenty-four hours on a keyboard.

- By themselves, these germs may not be a big deal, but if you're eating while typing and get your fingers in your mouth, or rub your eyes or nose, you can see how even the simple keyboard could be a problem.

- Things that can carry germs, such as finger oil, food residue, drinks, and so on, also have the added negative effect of possibly gumming up your keyboard and making it work less efficiently over time.

So, here's how to keep your keys in top shape and keep yourself safe.

- Wipe down your keyboard regularly with disinfecting wipes or a Q-tip doused in sterilizing liquid, such as isopropyl alcohol. Just running these over the surface a few times a week will help.

- For a laptop, consider getting a rubber shield to cover the keyboard. These are thin layers that lay over an existing keyboard and are molded to it exactly. They often come in different colors and patterns. They're easy to clean with wipes or a cloth and have the added bonus of keeping dirt and food particles out of the keys.

- When your laptop is off or you unplug your desktop keyboard, turn it over and gently shake to remove any bits that have gotten stuck. For more difficult pieces, try using some compressed air. For most desktop computers, you can remove the keys, if you really want to get a better clean.

- Keep food and drink well away from your keyboard!

- Wash your hands regularly, since this will reduce the number of germs you are adding to the keyboard to begin with.

Regular cleanings of your keyboard will keep it more germ-free and even help it last longer.

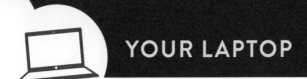

YOUR LAPTOP

Beyond just the keyboard itself, your laptop can host a whole number of germs and infectious things. The screen, the sides, the bottom—all can harbor hidden bacteria and infectious agents, especially if you take it out of your home frequently. At home, the same things apply as for other surfaces. And cats are notorious for loving the warmth of a good laptop, never mind what work you need to do!

- You open and close your laptop, take it with you, and handle it much more often than a desktop. All of this activity increases the chances of spreading germs to its surface.

- If you are using your laptop away from home, you'll be spreading whatever you pick up outside to it as you work, open and close it, etc. So even if you wash your hands when you get home, your laptop still has the germs you picked up outside.

- A laptop track pad is, as you might guess, a haven for germs, since our fingers drag across it all the time. It's comparable to a cell phone, and though it usually doesn't have nearly as many germs, it can still harbor some unpleasant things.

Cleaning a laptop doesn't have to be a huge chore, if you do a little bit every day. Here are some suggestions.

- Follow the same advice for your laptop keyboard cleaning as for a desktop. And use a rubber keyboard shield. Keeping dust out of your keyboard will also guard against the laptop overheating, potentially damaging the machine or draining the battery.

- Always turn off your laptop and unplug it before cleaning it.

- Clean off any initial dirt on the screen by gently wiping with a clean microfiber cloth.

- Never spray cleaners directly onto your laptop.

- Gently wipe down the screen and surface with a monitor-safe cleaner, preferably every day. This is important, because regular cleaners (even glass cleaners) can damage the screen. This will also help remove extra fingerprints and other residue. Never spray the device directly! Instead spray the cloth with a little cleaner and gently rub it over the glass surface. Let it air-dry.

- Close your laptop when it's off and keep it closed when not using it.

- After turning off your laptop and unplugging it, use disinfectant wipes or a damp cloth to regularly wipe down the top and bottom. Again, make sure these are computer safe.

These simple steps will keep your much-handled laptop in better shape and may help it last longer.

YOUR TABLET *and* OTHER DEVICES

You may already have some sense of just how germy your phone is; we'll get to that later on, and the truth is shocking! But if you use a tablet or an e-reader, the news isn't much better. In fact, since the screen is bigger on a tablet, it allows for that much more room for bacteria to take hold and grow. Wonderful! How dirty a tablet is depends on where it's been, how often you wash your hands, and how often you clean it.

- Studies have shown some tablets are great breeding grounds for staphylococcus aureus, the bacteria that cause staph infections. In fact, one study showed that the tablet had far more of these bacteria than the cell phone in the same study, and over thirty times as much as was found on a toilet seat!

- More research has revealed that a growing number of people view videos and other content on their tablets while in the bathroom, both at home and in public. This is just asking for germs to spread!

- Enterobacteria, which can cause everything from gastric problems to pneumonia, are another kind of bacteria commonly found on tablet surfaces.

So what to do when your supersized phone is a potential hazard? Here are some simple solutions.

- Wash your hands before and after using it. Always.

- Don't use devices on the toilet. Even if it's a great way to pass the time, leave them. This is even more the case when using public toilets, since you're touching handles and doorknobs that countless other hands (many unwashed) have also touched.

- Wipe down the surface with a lint-free cloth, such as the types used for cleaning eyeglasses. Do this every time you use the device.

- Clean the surface regularly, using a 70 percent ethanol or isopropyl alcohol solution. Wipes are the most convenient way to do this. Just make sure the device is off when you wipe it down! And be careful not to get any of the alcohol into the cracks where it could cause damage to the tablet itself. Focus on the glass surface only.

- Alcohol wipes are less desirable on an e-reader with a keyboard or other buttons, so be careful; you don't want to damage the device. Use a lint-free cloth instead, and as with other tablets, wash your hands before handling and using them.

Tablets are really just giant phones, and can be bigger breeding grounds for germs, but these simple steps will help reduce the risk of spreading them around.

VIDEO GAME CONTROLLERS *and* CONSOLES

Video game controllers, like TV remotes, are breeding grounds for just about everything you can imagine. We handle them frequently, often with dirty or food-covered hands, and pretty soon, various little microscopic nasties are popping up on them and transferring to and from our hands every time we play a game.

- Again, because we use them constantly, germs have the chance to build up, meaning controllers and consoles must be cleaned often.

- Dust, sweat, and other substances can also collect on them if they're not cleaned. These can also damage the controller and make it work less well over time.

- Controllers have been found to have seven times more germs on them than toilet seats.

- These numbers can get even worse if the player is sick, hasn't washed their hands, etc.

Video games are as much a part of our lives as TV and other entertainment, enjoyed by millions from age three to ninety-three, but kids especially love to play them, and kids can also be germ magnets. So, what can we do to keep our controllers cleaner and safer?

- Dust your controller and console regularly. They will collect dust when not being used, like anything else, so keep them dust-free. Consider storing the controller in a container or drawer where it will be less likely to get dusty. Cover your console with a cloth or other protective material. Just make sure that it is off and not in sleep mode, or it could overheat with a covering on it.

- Use disinfecting wipes, or a dedicated controller cleaner, at least once a week. Be mindful of buttons. Q-tips can work to get around areas more precisely.

- Be aware of foods and drink while you're playing. Gamers often love to eat while playing their favorite games, but this can get the controller dirtier and grubbier much faster. Sticky surfaces will attract even more germs. If you want to eat, try to eat things that are less likely to leave a mess on your controller.

All of this advice goes double if you have children. Keep their devices safe, and you'll all be happier!

In the age of streaming and downloading, CDs, DVDs, and Blu-Rays may be going the way of the dinosaurs, but millions of people still own them, use them, and love them. Discs of any kind are prone to getting worn out, whether they are for movies, music, or games. And even if you're careful when handling them, you still have to touch them. All of which means that they can get dirty and need to be kept clean. Here are some tips for ensuring they stay germ-free and have long lives. If you keep them long enough, they may even come back into fashion again!

- Discs of all kinds are just as susceptible to germs and bacteria as anything else in the home, so handle accordingly. Wash your hands before using and don't touch the playing surfaces, only the edges.

- Clean discs with a lint-free cloth, such as one made for eyeglasses. Do this regularly, preferably after each use/play, to get rid of any smudges and fingerprints. Clean both the side with writing, labels, and the playing side.

- Don't wipe discs in a circular motion; this can scratch the playing surface.

- Start in the middle hole and gently wipe straight out to the edge. Go around the disc until the whole surface is clean.

- If you need to get a better clean or if you've been sick, you can use a disc-cleaning solution (available at stores), or a lint-free cloth dampened with a bit of rubbing alcohol. In a pinch, take a small spoon of some mild soap and mix it into water. Dampen the cloth in the soapy water and use it to clean the disc. None of these cleaners will harm the disc's surface, but be sure to be gentle when cleaning. If you scrub too vigorously, you risk scratching the surface.

- If you use liquid to clean the disc, use a separate lint-free cloth to dry it off. Don't dry it off with paper products (towels, tissues, etc.), as these can be abrasive and leave small fibers behind on the surface.

- Always store your discs in their original cases. Never stack them up unprotected or leave them lying around, especially with the playing side facing down. This will ensure they stay dust, scratch, and germ-free. Discs will inevitably acquire some scratches over time, but most of these won't affect playback, as long as they are minor. All the more reason to keep them in their proper storage containers between uses!

If you're determined to hang on to your discs, then keep them clean, and they'll last you for years!

BOOKS

Most of us have at least a few books on shelves in our home; some of us have a lot more than that! Book lovers and book collectors take great pride in their hoard, whether they're antiques or just the latest paperbacks. But how safe are they? It would seem reasonable to think that, like anything else in the home, books could gather bacteria and viruses. And they can, but the risk seems to be low. So, if you're worried about books carrying all sorts of contagions, you can relax a little; but what about new books you've just bought, or, library books?

Library books would seem to be a potential source of infections. If multiple people are handling and retuning them, won't those germs build up over time? Studies have shown that even in this case, the risk is pretty small. Viruses only stay active on book surfaces for about twelve hours, so even if someone with the flu sneezed on a book and returned it the same day, the chances of someone else picking up that flu are small; it would likely sit for some time before reshelving, unless there was an immediate demand for it. If you love your library, here are some things to remember.

- You're unlikely to get sick from handling library books. Tests have found small traces of harmful bacteria and such on various books, but the amounts are usually too small to be worried about.

- If germs are something you are concerned about, when you get home, you can quarantine books (see below). If a book has a plastic cover, you can wipe it down with an disinfecting wipe; just be sure not to get any liquid onto the cover or the book's pages!

- It's more likely than an older book may have dust, fungi, or other allergens on it. If you haunt used-book stores, and you're subject to allergies, you might want to bear that in mind. But again, unless you're holding the book up to your nose and inhaling for a good length of time, you probably won't be affected. You can try setting a musty book in direct sunlight for a few days, but don't leave it there indefinitely, as sunlight will fade colors on books over time.

- Studies are ongoing about how much, if any, bacteria can persist on a book's cover or pages, but so far, it doesn't seem to be a high risk. This is true even with COVID-19. But if you want to be absolutely sure, place any books you bring into your home in a dedicated place for twenty-four hours, and don't touch them before that time period has passed. Yes, that may be too difficult to contemplate if it's a book you really need to read!

Books are treasures, and thankfully, they don't seem to be a big problem when it comes to spreading disease. But keep them well-dusted and clean on their shelves in any case!

WINDOWS

Windows are made of glass, and like any surface, viruses and bacteria can be found on them. Thankfully, keeping them clean is not a difficult job.

- There were some early concerns that COVID-19 could live on glass surfaces for up to four days. However, as with other surfaces, this is far more likely if an infected person coughs or sneezes on the window glass, and someone else immediately touches the surface and then rubs their eyes or nose. In short, it's possible, but not that likely.

- Still, any kind of virus, such as a cold or flu virus, can find its way onto a window and hang out there for a while.

- Dirty windows can block as much as 40 percent of natural outside light from getting in. If you suffer from Seasonal Affective Disorder (SAD) or similar concerns, having clean windows can make a huge difference to your mood.

To remedy this:

- Clean your windows often. Start by brushing or sweeping to remove dust and cobwebs.

- Use a good commercial glass cleaner, or one that you've made yourself. White vinegar is a great all-purpose cleaner. Mix one part white vinegar to one part hot water and use a sponge, squeegee, or spray bottle. Use a cloth or even newspaper to get your windows squeaky clean and streak-free!

- Don't clean a window when the sun is directly shining on it. The heat can make your cleaning solution dry too quickly, leaving streaks on the glass.

- Rinse off and dry the window frames to avoid damaging them.

- Keep your windows open when you're home, if the weather permits it. Even in winter, a little bit every day will help. An open window lets fresh air circulate and reduces the chances of infection, as contaminated air is recycled out and replaced with fresher air. Viruses, including COVID-19, do not randomly waft along in the outside air, so you're not in danger of inviting in any infections when leaving your window open. Even just having two windows open for a few minutes is enough to circulate the air.

Windows won't likely be a major source of concern when it comes to germs, but cleaning them regularly and opening them frequently can play an important role in reducing contaminants of all kinds.

CHILDREN'S TOYS

If anything is going to be a germ magnet in your home, it's children's toys! Whether plush or plastic, these treasured objects will be subjected to a lot of love . . . and spit and snot and unwashed hands. Keeping them clean is essential for your children's health and the household's.

- Children are more than twice as likely to get sick during cold and flu season as adults, and an easy way for viruses to take up residence in your home is through their toys.

- Bacteria can live on both hard and soft surfaces and be spread around as soon as your kids use one toy and then move onto another.

- Other nasties, such as lice and pinworms, love to find their way to where children are, and hitch a ride on hair, skin, and clothing.

- Pink eye, whether viral or bacterial, is a scourge of classrooms, and can easily be transferred from one child to another if one rubs the eyes, touches a toy, and then hands it on to another child.

- Indeed, toys taken to school can pick up all kinds of things, especially if they're shared.

- Soft toys can also collect dust mites, like mattresses and pillows, which can make allergies worse.

Here are some easy and useful tips for keeping your kids' beloved objects safer and healthier.

- Make sure your children wash their hands as soon as they get home, before picking up anything. This is especially true if they're just home from school and have been around dozens of other incubators of whatever might be going around! Clean hands are always one of the best ways to stop the spread of germs.

- For video games, see the game controller entry above.

- Hard toys can be disinfected with wipes regularly. Some of them might be suitable to wash with soap and warm water, or even to go in the dishwasher, but be sure to check first, so you don't accidentally destroy a favorite item!

- Soft toys are often machine washable, and can go in the dryer, too. Check the tag for information. Washing every other week is a good idea. Don't use bleach and follow the tag's instructions, if there are any.

- If a soft toy can't go in the machine, gently hand-washing the surface with a mild soap will usually do the trick. Take a washcloth and clean the whole surface, taking care not to soak the toy. Let it dry in the sun.

- Another good trick for hand-washed soft toys is to put them in a plastic freezer bag and store them in your freezer for three days. This will kill remaining germs. Just bear in mind that not having their favorite stuffed toy for three days could be difficult for your child, so plan accordingly.

Keeping toys clean is an ongoing task, but one that will help your kids (and you!) stay healthier.

THE DINING ROOM *and* KITCHEN TABLES

Your food tables get a lot of use, and it's easy for germs, dust, and food bits to build up on them quickly. Pretty much every bacteria or virus that can be found in your home will also end up where you eat, yuck!

- Glass and wooden surfaces are natural places for germs to congregate, especially tabletops, where people gather often and eat (and spill!) food. Damp spots will encourage bacterial growth.

- Unwashed hands are a major culprit in the spread of germs at mealtime.

Here's how to keep your eating spaces cleaner.

- Always wash your hands before eating, even if you've been at home. This goes for everyone in the house.

- Glass tabletops can be cleaned daily or every other day. Wipe down first with a slightly damp cloth and then apply the spray and clean as you would normally, wiping the surface dry.

- Clean a wooden table by first wiping it down. A slightly damp microfiber cloth is great, because it collects more dust, crumbs, and other debris. Wipe down your tables with one of these every day, or every other day. Follow this at least once a week by using a cloth wetted with a cleaning solution, either store-bought, or a mixture of two to three cups of warm water and a few drops of dishwashing soap. A mixture of one part water to one part white vinegar is also a great cleaner.

- Buff the table dry after cleaning. Commercial dusting sprays are not necessary and over time, they can lead to a buildup of even more dust and dirt.

- If you have a cloth tablecloth, wash it regularly (once a week), as spills, stains, and germs will build up on it. Many are machine washable. If your table covering is made of something other than cloth, follow any instructions on how to clean. A simple plastic or vinyl covering can be easily wiped down and cleaned on a regular basis.

- If you have a major food or drink spill, try to clean it as soon as you can. Don't leave it to sink into cloth or sit on a wooden surface.

Keeping your dining tables clean is easy and shouldn't take a lot of time. Since these are the focus of your meals, you need to keep them as clean as possible!

SALT AND PEPPER SHAKERS, *and* OTHER HANDHELD OBJECTS

You'll obviously wash your utensils with each use, but a surprising number of food items and tools are used and reused without thinking about how dirty they might get: salt and pepper shakers, vinegar bottles, oil bottles, water pitchers, etc. It doesn't make a lot of sense to keep your table clean and your hands well washed, if you're going to be handling the same dirty salt shaker day after day!

- Any items that you don't clean up will retain germs on their surfaces. If you go days or weeks without cleaning them, this will only get worse. Unfortunately, some people never bother to clean them.

- Objects like salt and pepper shakers tend to be brought out, used, and stored again (or left on the table) without ever being washed off. It's not something we usually think about, probably because our actual contact with them is minimal. But germs transfer quickly.

- Coliform bacteria and even E. coli can take up residence on items near food that aren't cleaned properly and regularly. That means that even if you've washed your hands, if you pick up a water pitcher or salt shaker that has these bacteria, you'll be potentially transferring them to your utensils and food in short order.

Fortunately, it's not difficult to cut down on germs around your food, provided you do it regularly.

- Wash your hands before every meal. This should be obvious, but it's amazing how often people forget to do it, or just don't think it's important. It is important. The germs that collect on glass, wood, and plastic surfaces will be the ones that you and others are bringing with them, so don't being them with you to begin with!

- Clean these items regularly with disinfecting wipes or a bit of rubbing alcohol and a cloth. If something is made of wood (such as a pepper grinder), clean it in the same way you would clean a wooden table: rub it down with a damp cloth regularly, and once a week or so, clean the surface with some water and a few drops of dishwashing liquid or a one part water to one part vinegar solution.

- If your items are dishwasher-safe, empty out the contents (salt, pepper, etc.) into a temporary container and give their homes a good machine wash once every few weeks. The hot water and detergent will sterilize them. Just make sure they are thoroughly dried before putting contents back into them!

These kinds of containers are easy to overlook when cleaning your home and dining spaces, so make sure to give them the same good cleaning you would for anything else that comes into contact with food.

OTHER HOUSEHOLD FURNITURE

Beyond dining tables, your home is filled with furniture that has all kinds of surfaces—wood, glass, cloth—that can easily attract and retain germs. Every time you touch something, sit on a chair, or flop on the couch, you're picking up bacteria and spreading it around. Other common substances around the home include yeast and various molds.

- **Chairs:** For wooden chairs, clean like you would a wooden table. For a chair that has a cloth cushion, check to see if it is detachable and machine washable. If not, follow the guidelines for sofas.

- **Sofas:** Sofas are places that we, our children, and our pets love to lounge on, and that means that they are prime attractors of germs. For a quick clean, use a stiff, dry brush to remove hair and grit. Go over the entire surface of the couch. Use a vacuum to suck up ground-in dirt and hair. Try using baking soda. Sprinkle over the entirety of the couch, gently rub in, and wait fifteen to twenty minutes before vacuuming it off. It will help remove odors and stains.

- **Filthy sofas:** Check the sofa tag for the manufacturer's cleaning code. *W* means water-based cleaners only, *S/W* means solvents and water-based cleaners, while *S* means solvents-only. *X* means no liquids at all, vacuum-only. Make sure you are using the right cleaner to spot-clean your sofa! Gently dry with a towel and let the surface air-dry completely before putting back pillows or coverings.

- **Doorknobs and stair rails:** Our hands touch these all the time, so be sure to wipe them down with disinfectant (in wipes or a spray with a cloth) at least once a week. If you have guests over, be sure to clean when they've gone.

- **Desks and end tables:** Wipe down work areas, nightstands, and so on with a lint-free cloth or a commercial duster every few days. As with wood tables, commercial dusting sprays are not advisable, because they build up over time. At most, a slightly damp cloth should be enough to keep the surface clean and grit-free.

- **Bookcases:** Regular dusting will keep your books and display objects cleaner, and not allow allergens and dust bunnies to build up. If you have glass-covered cases, this will go a long way to keeping the contents cleaner. Just clean the glass as you would a window, and dust inside once in a while.

- **TV cases:** As with a bookcase, a TV center can trap dust all over it. Keeping dust from building up here will not only keep your home cleaner, but also it will save wear and tear on your electronic devices, and prevent damage to internal hardware. Use a slightly damp microfiber cloth to wipe dust from your flat screen TV; be gentle! It will keep the surface clean and improve picture quality.

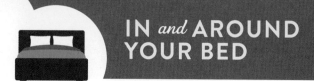

IN *and* AROUND YOUR BED

Beds and pillows can be one of the worst places for attracting bacteria, viruses, and dust mites. It's inevitable that a place where we spend about a third of our lives will be a breeding ground for bacteria. What's on our bodies will transfer to the bed, and what's on the bed will transfer to us.

- Dust mites are a thing. They are in your bed. They thrive in dusty environments and their waste (yes, their poop!) can cause allergic reactions, sometimes severe ones.

- Certain types of moths thrive in dust. Their larvae can hatch from eggs in spaces behind and under beds.

- One study of pillows showed that they had forty-seven types of fungi and mold in them! The most common type found was *aspergillus fumigatus*, which can cause all kinds of health problems in immune-compromised people.

- Bacteria from our bodies and sweat build up over night and stay on the sheets after we get up. If you have staph or strep on your skin, it could infect anyone else sleeping in the bed.

Obviously, keeping your bedroom clean is a must. Here's how.

- Wash your bedsheets and pillowcases once a week in hot water, or at least warm water. If someone in your home is sick, wash more frequently. Wash blankets and duvets regularly.

- Consider washing your bedroom laundry separately from other clothing, especially anything with outside dirt on it.

44

- Don't eat in bed. Sorry to say, it will only attract more bacteria and maybe even pests, such as ants, fleas, bedbugs, and dust mites.

- Run a lint roller over your duvet each day to remove hair and dust—especially if you have pets.

- Get dust mite–proof covers for your pillows. Or even whole pillows that are dust mite–proof (yes, they exist and work well!).

- Don't let your bedroom get too warm or humid. Mites thrive in those environments, and can't breed as well when the temperature falls below 77°F.

- Consider getting an air purifier for the bedroom. These machines can circulate air and remove particles (dust and spores).

- Open the windows when the weather is good, and let that fresh air circulate! Even a few minutes will do a room good. Air quality has become more of a concern in recent years for many, especially those living in fire-prone areas. When the air quality index is 50 or below, it is considered good and having your windows open is recommended. If the number goes above that, it's better to keep them closed. There are many apps and websites that track local air quality.

IN YOUR CLOSETS
and DRESSERS

Closets and clothing drawers aren't huge havens for bacteria, unless you live in a humid environment. Still, it's nice to keep them clean. The declutter movement that has become popular in the last few years has given many people ideas about how to simplify their lives, but there's also been a backlash against it, with some thinking that it goes too far. Whichever side you're on, it's still obvious that your closets and drawers need to be kept clean.

• Overstuffed closets can become havens for dust and can attract dust mites and moths. If you live in a humid area, mold growth is also a possibility. This can lead to musty smells that permeate your clothes. Dampness can also encourage the growth of odor-causing bacteria.

• Dust is less likely in drawers that remain closed most of the time, but your clothes can still attract moths and other insects.

Here are some useful tips for keeping these areas clean, as well as pest, and mold-free.

• Never put dirty clothes back into a drawer or closet. That's just asking for bad smells and bacteria growth! Have a dedicated clothes basket for everything that needs to be washed.

• For a regular deep clean of your closet, remove everything. Yes everything! You're going to want to get into cracks and crevices, and you don't want hanging clothes getting in your way.

• Use a lightly damp cloth to wipe away extra dust and grime. Use a mild household all-purpose cleaner to remove any stains or spots.

- Pay attention to the walls and ceilings, too. You may need a broom to sweep away cobwebs.

- Be sure to dry off every surface afterward, so that there won't be any dampness left over that could seep into your clothes.

- If your closet floor is carpeted, sprinkle some baking soda on it and let it sit for fifteen to twenty minutes before vacuuming it up. This will help eliminate any musty smells or other undesirable odors.

- As long as you already have everything out, now is a good time to take stock of everything and see if you really need it all. Clearing out your clutter a bit can make it easier to keep clean and reduce the chance of messes in the future.

- Use garment bags for your best items, to keep them safe.

- Use silica gel packets or other moisture absorbers (scented or unscented) for any areas in the closet that might get damp.

- Clean your drawers in a similar way: remove all clothes and wipe down the drawers to remove dust and grit. Wait until your drawers are completely dry before putting your clothes back in.

- Cedar chips and blocks are a great moth repellent; use them in your drawers and closets. Scented natural potpourri bags and sachets are also a good way of keeping things smelling fresh.

YOUR DRAPES
and CARPETS

Carpets are obviously a potential hazard in the home. Most homes have them, but they're great for trapping bacteria, germs, hair, outside dirt, pet fluff, food crumbs, and just about anything else you can imagine! You might be surprised to learn that curtains are not much better. Because they're hanging up and out of the way, we tend to ignore them, even during regular cleanings. This can be a mistake.

- As with other fabrics, drapes and curtains can accumulate dust and dust mites, along with many other allergens. If you're finding that you have allergies that seem worse when you're at home, your curtains and carpets may be to blame.

- If anyone is sick and virus particles are circulating through the house, they can easily land on curtains. So can bacteria from outside.

- And with carpets, the story is even worse: they can harbor up 4,000 times more bacteria per square inch than a toilet seat! Just think about everything that falls on your floor every day, and this makes sense.

- Carpets also attract dust mites, and a clean-looking carpet can actually have up to one pound of dirt per yard, ground in and invisible!

- Mold likes carpets, too.

- Some viruses can live for days or even weeks in your carpet.

- Knowing all this, you really should abandon the "five second rule" about dropped food. Seriously. Germs and other nasty things will happily stick to your food instantly.

Wow, OK, so what should you do? Don't panic!

- Dust your curtains and try using a roller for anything (hair, dirt, etc.) that's stuck on. If they are washable, wash them every few months. If not, consider dry cleaning them.

- Always take your outdoor shoes off at the door and store them in a dedicated space. Don't walk on your carpets with outside shoes.

- Remember that a carpet actually works well as a kind of air filter. Dirt, dust, germs, and other things get pulled down and trapped in it. That's good for you and the air you breathe, but not so good for the carpet!

- Clean up after pets as soon as possible.

- Use a carpet sweeper daily, if you have one, and vacuum at least once a week.

- This kind of regular carpet cleaning will certainly help, but a good steam cleaning will pull much more dirt (and everything else!) out of the carpet. Steam cleaning is often best done by professionals and is something you should consider once or twice a year.

Carpets and curtains present a challenge to keeping your home safe from bacteria, viruses, and more, but with some planning, you can keep them much cleaner than they probably are right now.

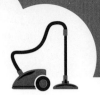

YOUR VACUUM CLEANER

The vacuum cleaner is one of your chief weapons in the war on germs, but it might not have occurred to you that it can get dirty and "germy" too! Vacuums are pretty much essential to modern cleaning, but they can cause their own problems too.

- Vacuums are great, even necessary, but they can actually blow germs and bacteria around your house while you're cleaning! How fun! It really depends on the quality of the machine you have. The better the filter, the more it will trap and prevent from scattering. However, studies have shown that even HEPA filters don't always work as well as they should (or as some people say they do!).

- The older the machine, the worse this spreading of particles will be. If you're using one from twenty years ago, it's probably making you sick.

- An Australian study concluded: "Both vacuum cleaning and the act of vacuuming can release and re-suspend dust and allergens, leading to increased exposure."

- Bacteria such as salmonella and E. coli have been found growing inside bags and chambers.

So, should we stop vacuuming completely? Of course not! But what do we do?

- Keep on vacuuming. It's infinitely better than not doing it at all!

- Invest in a good, new vacuum cleaner. There really is no other choice. Whether you use a traditional bag variety, or a bagless model, the better the quality, the more it will pick up from your floors, and the less likely it will be to spread around the same germs it's picking up.

- Dispose of bags promptly after use; don't let them sit in the machine.

- If you vacuum is bagless, empty it into a large plastic bag or an outside garbage container after each use. You may want to wear a mask if dust clouds go flying about.

- Clean the machine itself. Wipe it down with some disinfectant wipes or a damp cloth and some spray on the cloth. If anything from inside has settled on the outside, you can wipe it off.

- Keep the brushes clean. They can capture hair and dust clumps that can slow them down. Wearing a latex (or non rubber) glove, pull out any hairs and other debris caught in the brushes.

- If you have a bagless machine, clean the inside chamber regularly with a bit of diluted bleach (one part bleach to ten parts water) or soap and water, after you've removed the washable parts. Always wear gloves!

The vacuum is an essential tool to keeping things clean, but make sure you don't neglect to keep it clean and safe, too!

IN YOUR WASHING MACHINE

Here's some bad news: the one place that you would think would be free of germs actually has a lot! A washing machine regularly sees soap and water, so what's the problem? Well, the machine can pick up any contaminants from clothing, and if there are plastic surfaces inside the machine (and most have them), these bacteria and other germs will often take up residence. And in the damp environment of the machine, they will only grow and multiply!

So, before we get into taking better care of your laundry, what can you do to help disinfect your machine?

- Clean your washing machine regularly. This doesn't have to be a big task, just get in there and scrub out the drum the way you would for any household surface. Use a commercial cleaner, or equal parts hot water and vinegar, or even baking soda.

- Clean the detergent drawer. Take it out and soak it in warm water with a bit of soap (such as dishwashing liquid) for fifteen to twenty minutes. Clean out the space where it sits while you're letting it soak. A toothbrush is great for this. Clean the drawer out with more soap and water after it's soaked. A separate toothbrush is great for this, too. Let it air-dry before putting it back in the space.

- Clean the machine's rubber seal with some soap and warm water. Don't use any stronger cleaners, as this can erode the seal over time and cause your machine to leak.

- For other areas, such as the filter or drainpipe, consult your machine's manual for instructions.

- Place soda crystals or washing machine cleaning tablets in the drum and run the machine without clothes on the hottest cycle available. Do this once a month. Some machines have instructions on doing a maintenance wash to keep things running smoothly and to keep the machine cleaner.

- Try to do one hot wash a week. This will kill bacteria and help prevent their growth.

- Clean out your dryer's lint catcher after every use (a fire safety issue), and also gently clean the inside periodically, as you would the washing machine drum. Again, make sure to let it dry completely before using.

These simple steps will reduce the amount of bacteria in your washing machine, and keep it from spreading to your nice, clean clothes, which, if you don't clean the machine, really aren't so clean after all!

YOUR LAUNDRY

There are scads of nasty microorganisms parading around in your dirty clothes.

- Studies have shown all kinds of bacteria can live in machines and dirty clothes, including E. coli, salmonella, staphylococcus. E.coli in particular grows well in damp towels.

- The bacteria from one load of laundry can remain in the machine and contaminate future loads.

- Cold water washes save energy but can often be ineffective at getting rid of germs. Warm is better and hot is the best.

- Clothes that smell bad may or may not have dangerous bacteria, so there's no "smell test" to determine it.

So, what to do? Thankfully, the solutions are easy!

- Don't let dirty clothes sit in the clothes hamper for days, much less weeks. This will just give bacteria more time to multiply, making them a lot worse. Shuffle clothes in and out of it regularly.

- Wash clothes that permit it in hot water. The higher the temperature, the more germs the water will kill. Of course, some delicates and fabrics need cold water, so be sure not to mix them into your hot water loads. They can be hand-washed separately.

- Use a detergent with bleach to kill germs. Be careful with certain colors or fabrics; you may need to wash them separately. Look for a bleach that has a hydrogen peroxide (H_2O_2) base; it's less likely to strip color from clothes. And check all your clothing's tags for specific instructions!

- Wash underwear separately. Fecal matter is in most underwear, and the bacteria in it can contaminate other clothing in the same load.

- Wash children's clothing separately. These items can pick up many germs from their various daily travels and adventures, and especially during cold season, it's a good idea to isolate kid's clothing.

- Wash towels separately. Since they get damp more often, they will be breeding grounds for all kinds of invisible things. Also, change out your towels often, and don't use them if they're still damp from previous use. Let them dry out completely.

- Wash your hands after handling dirty laundry, or you'll spread germs around. Wash them again after moving wet laundry to the dryer.

- Dry clothing on the medium setting at least, and on hot if the fabric permits it. Dry for at least forty-five minutes, or longer.

- When the weather permits, dry your clothes outside on a line, in the sun. The UV light from the sun acts as a natural disinfectant and will kill extra bacteria that may still be on your clothes. Just be mindful of outside pollens. You could be trading bacteria for allergens!

- Periodically sanitize your clothes hamper with a disinfectant spray. Make sure that it's dried out completely before putting in more clothes.

THE FIREPLACE

Germs in your fireplace? Yes! Above and beyond other safety concerns, such as keeping the chimney clean and sweeping out ash, a fireplace can harbor just as many germs and bacteria as anywhere else in your house. And if you don't use it regularly, it can be worse.

- If you're not using your fireplace, it can sometimes become a haven for nesting birds or other small animals that can bring bacteria, pests, and other infectious agents with them.

- The ash and soot that collects in the fireplace can harbor all kinds of allergens and potentially toxic compounds.

- Anything that collects in the fireplace can be tracked into your living room, especially if you don't have a glass screen in front of it.

Cleaning a chimney may seem laborious, but you probably won't have to do it as often, unless you use your fireplace quite a lot.

- Only clean after at least twelve hours have passed since your previous fire.

- Have a professional chimney sweeping service check your fireplace each year before you use it.

- Have the flue checked for bird's nests and other intrusions, including looking for animal feces and droppings. If these have fallen into your fireplace, they could be breeding grounds for all kinds of bacteria.

- Make sure the surrounding area is well covered and have a plastic bag at hand to collect ash and soot. Wear old clothes and gloves (preferably rubber gloves). Wear a dust mask to protect yourself, and goggles if you need to.

- Remove all ash and dust with a hand broom and a dustpan. Sweep ash and dust off the grate, and then take it outside to clean. A commercial cleaner or soap and hot water should do the trick. Leave to air-dry.

- Use a dry bristle brush to scrape down the sides of the fireplace, as high as you can reach.

- Do a deeper clean. Use a commercial all-purpose cleaning spray or a homemade one, such as a half cup of bleach in a bucket of hot water, and wash down the insides and floor. If you have an older fireplace, be careful not to scrub too hard. Dry off with a cloth or towel that's disposable, and let it finish by air-drying.

A chimney may not be the first place you'd think of to fight germs, but keeping it clean and inspected can help prevent outside contaminants from getting in.

HIDDEN DUST PILES

In the course of your cleaning, it's inevitable that you'll miss some places, or probably won't want to be bothered to get everywhere. A "good enough" cleaning usually is, but if you do too many of those in a row, dust, dirt, and germs can really build up. This is especially true of those hidden places we never really think about.

Some of the prime examples include:

- **Under the bed:** especially if you also use the space under your bed for storage. When you pull out everything, you'll be shocked at how much dust has accumulated. And in that dust can live dust mites, moth larvae, and unknown amounts of bacteria.

- **Behind the bed:** where the frame meets the wall. If you haven't looked back there in a while, you'll be astonished by how dusty and dirty it is!

- **Under dressers:** if you have dressers and chests that are elevated off the floor by short legs, it's guaranteed that dust bunnies and other things will collect under there. They can be prime breeding grounds for moths and other creatures.

- **Houseplants:** they add beauty to your home, but they can collect dust, shed particles, and spread dirt easily. Be sure to take good care of them and keep the area around them clean. Dust the leaves regularly, and keep an eye out for pests and infections.

- **The tops of bookcases:** just because you can't see them or reach them doesn't mean they're not getting dirty! Huge amounts of dust can gather up there over time, and it's worth getting on a ladder or chair once a month or so to keep them clean.

- **The tops of books, video games, CDs, and DVDs:** lots of dust piles up in these locations, so run a duster over them as you clean, preferably one that grips dust and holds it. Feather dusters just spread dust and everything in it around!

- **The tops of kitchen shelves:** if your cabinetry doesn't go all the way to the ceiling, or if you have extra shelving that's exposed to the air, dirt and grime are already there.

- **Shelving for TVs and stereos:** it's easy to forget about the small spaces behind these, especially if, for example, you have a large TV screen set into a cabinet or mounted on a wall. But dust will collect in these places as easily as anywhere, so be sure to give them an occasional clean.

These areas can collect dust quickly, and with it, dust mites, moths, and other pests, along with pollen, other allergens, and dangerous bacteria. Be sure to make the effort to clean them at least once a month. A vacuum extension or a hand vacuum will usually do the trick. If it's especially bad (and we've all left these areas for too long), you may need to also clean the area with a damp cloth to remove any ground-in dirt or grime that has accumulated.

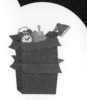

IN THE BASEMENT

Basements are natural collectors of all things related to dirt and germs, and often we ignore that fact (or pretend to!) for far too long, until the idea of cleaning it seems overwhelming. And if it is overwhelming, you may have to do it in stages.

- One of the chief problems with basements is that they get damp, and when they do, they can be prime breeding grounds for all sorts of molds and bacteria. And if they travel through things likes HVAC ducts (and they do!), they can spread throughout the home, causing allergies and worse.

- Dust mites thrive in humid air. If your basement is dusty, they'll be there. They'll soon leave their cozy basement homes and travel into the house looking for food. And they'll leave droppings that cause allergic reactions.

- Rats and other small creatures find ways into basements quite easily. Many of them have ticks, or worse, fleas. Fleas multiply at an astonishing rate and can carry all kinds of disease. Remember the Black Death? The bubonic plague? It's a bacteria-caused illness from fleas and it's still a thing. People contract it every year.

- Rodents can also carry the dangerous hantavirus in their droppings. This can become airborne if the feces dry out enough, and can enter into your home, with potentially deadly consequences.

Clearly, you need to keep your basement clean! But it doesn't have to be a Herculean task.

- First, have your basement inspected by a professional. They'll look for leaks, damp patches, holes, damage, problems with your water heater, and anything else that could let in water, pests, and outside invaders. If there are any of these issues, you'll need to have the problems fixed by professionals.

- Once they've eliminated the bigger problems, it's an easier task to keep the basement relatively clean. Sweep it out regularly, and don't let dust or cobwebs accumulate. Wear a mask.

- If you have a lot of junk stored down there, go through it and get rid of what you don't need; there's probably a lot that can be thrown out or donated, sold, etc. Do this in stages so it doesn't feel overwhelming. Store what you do keep in a more orderly fashion, preferably in waterproof, plastic containers.

- Once the floor is cleared and swept, you'll probably want to mop, to remove extra dirt. Soap and a bucket of warm water should do the trick, though a dedicated floor cleaner is fine, too. Be sure to let the floor dry completely before putting anything back.

- Consider buying some damp ridder packets to take excess moisture out of the air. There are also air fresheners that reduce moldy and musty smells.

- Sweep regularly to keep down dust, and check for anything like animal droppings or chew marks.

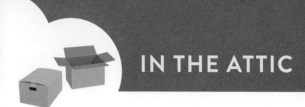

IN THE ATTIC

Like basements, attics are breeding grounds for all sorts of infectious things, especially if you rarely use yours, and throw things up there in storage for months or years at a time. Rats, squirrels, possums, and other small animals absolutely love attics and crawl spaces, so there's a good chance that sooner or later, some of them will take up residence above you. And the same problems that you face in the basement will also be present up there: potentially contaminated droppings, fleas, urine sprays, and dust, hair, and dust mites.

So, what to do?

- As with your basement, have your attic professionally inspected. They can look for infestations of rats and other pests, and create solutions that will eliminate them, as well as checking for mold and dampness problems. They can also advise you on the state of your insulation.

- Your attic might need more cleaning afterward. Be careful about rodent droppings and urine. Don't just sweep them up. Instead, spray urine and feces with a mixture of one part bleach to ten parts water, and let it soak for at least five minutes.

- Wearing a mask and rubber gloves, use paper towels to wipe up sprays and pick up droppings. Dispose of them in a plastic bag. Make sure to disinfect your gloves and clothing afterward.

- If any of your boxes or other storage materials have become contaminated, remove them outside and disinfect in the sunlight, if you can.

- Always store your items in sealed plastic containers. Cardboard can easily become contaminated, damp, chewed on, and so on. If you have anything stored in cardboard boxes, some items may have been ruined by an infestation. Remove them carefully to outdoors and examine them while wearing gloves. Glass, plastic, and metal objects can usually be washed and disinfected. With paper, it's less likely. Be careful what you store up there and how you store it!

- Once your attic is cleaned and dried out, keep it clean with regular sweepings and dustings. If you can take a vacuum up there, do so.

- If your attic is only a crawl space, it can still be subject to invasions by rats and other creatures. You may not be able to fit comfortably into it. Use a professional cleaning service to eliminate the problem and disinfect the area.

The attic needs to become a part of your cleaning routine, and if you keep at it, you and your possessions will be much happier!

IN YOUR GARAGE

One other "added on" area to most houses is the garage, which, although intended for your car, often becomes a catch-all storage unit for anything that doesn't fit elsewhere. This is just asking for trouble. Remember that your car (like the soles of your shoes) is out on roads and in parking lots, and its tires are potentially picking up all sorts of bacteria (among other things), and wheeling it back to your garage, where it can take up residence.

Keeping your garage clean will go a long way toward preventing outside contaminants from getting into your home to begin with. Here are some tips.

- As with your basement and attic, your garage may be more than just messy. If you have any kind of infestation, you may need professional help to clear it up. It's best to have it checked out if you see anything out of sorts.

- Once you're sure that you've eliminated rodents, cockroaches, and other unwanted guests, you can begin to clean the garage in the same way you did the basement and attic: take everything out (including your car!) and be ready to toss or donate things you no longer use, want, or need.

- If anything is damaged, clean or disinfect it using the guidelines for the basement and attic. Some items may be damaged beyond repair.

- Wearing a mask, sweep and dust the area to remove excess debris, cobwebs, and anything else that might be lingering around. A push broom is great for this kind of cleaning, but a regular one will do just fine.

- After the sweeping, it's time to mop! Follow the instructions for cleaning your basement and get that garage floor nice and washed! Allow it to dry completely before moving your car back in.

- Some people recommend painting your garage floor. It helps seal out moisture and prolong the life of the floor. It's up to you, but it might be a good investment. Look for one-part epoxy paint specifically made for garage floors, as it resists mold, gas stains, scuffing, and wearing out better than other paints.

- Make a reorganization plan for the things you need to keep. Consider using plastic storage containers and put long-term storage items where you won't reach them as easily. The things you use more often can then be placed on top or in front of them, or wherever is most convenient.

- Make cleaning your garage a part of your regular cleaning routine, at least once every other week. A little bit every time keeps it from becoming a bigger and less appealing job.

The garage is an important side-room to most houses, so make sure yours is as germ-free as possible and usable for more than just being a place to park your car.

CHAPTER 2:
GERMS IN THE KITCHEN

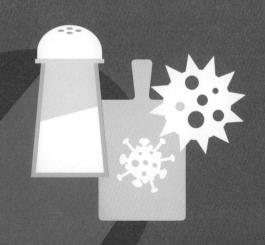

For many (most?), the kitchen is the most important place in the home. It's where all of our beloved food and drinks are, so naturally, we want to go there often. Unfortunately, germs think so, too! It's probably no surprise to you that the kitchen can be one of the germiest places in the house, since bacteria from all kinds of foods can hitch a ride in from outside and set up camp with ease. Food can also get shoved to the back of the refrigerator or cupboard, to be forgotten and left to grow exciting new colonies of experimental life!

Obviously, keeping your kitchen clean is essential to your good health. This chapter will detail some of the shocking and not-so-shocking places that germs can roam freely around your kitchen and on your food and give you plenty of ways to stop them from getting out of hand. It's your food, after all, not theirs!

THE REFRIGERATOR HANDLE

When you're in the kitchen, whether prepping for your holiday dinner or just getting a midnight snack, you're probably not thinking about all the germs that you're leaving and/or picking up from the handle of your refrigerator every time you open the door. But they're there, oh yes, they are (and just wait until you read about office refrigerators in chapter 4!). Keep in mind these points: As with so many of the items in your kitchen, door handles are great surfaces for allowing germs to collect and spread. They are touched frequently, even throughout the day, and if you have several people living in your home, each is bringing their own unique cocktail of germs with them whenever they touch this main portal to the food. That's not a great situation!

- Think about all the kinds of food that are stored in a refrigerator. These innocuous knobs can pretty quickly get covered with a combination of meat residue, spices, and milk products that create a recipe for bad microorganisms to thrive.

- Raw meat often contains fecal bacteria, which can easily end up on the door handle, only to hop onto your hand and then go on its merry way to some other part of your kitchen or home. A recent study showed that, in over 4,590 pounds of raw meat examined, *all* of it had some fecal contamination, and almost 20 percent had food poisoning bacteria. If you go and pick up a tomato or some salad leaves, guess what gets into them

- Even if you don't eat meat, various germs can still build up, just from regular use over time. This is especially true if someone is not as good about washing their hands as they should be, and then they go into the kitchen for a quick snack.

Fortunately, the fix is easy. Here's how to de-grossify that handle and keep those nasty germs from getting all over your hands and clean food:

- To avoid germs setting up an outpost outside your fridge, just make sure you wipe down the handle each time you clean the kitchen (even more often would be good). A commercial cleaner, or your own mix of one part vinegar to one part hot water will work just fine. Use a cloth and give it a good wipe.

- Be sure to clean underneath it and on the hinges, all those little areas that are easy to miss!

- Do this cleaning regularly, and you'll prevent bacteria from growing and building up. It's a good idea to at least wipe down the handle every time you've finished opening and closing the door, say, after dinner when you're bringing back dishes from the dinner table.

- You'll also make sure that you're not transferring undesirable invisible things from your raw meat or the outside world to everything else that you eat!

IN THE FRIDGE

It's not just issues with your food (we'll get to that in the next section); your refrigerator itself could be a problem for bacteria and other growing things you don't want in there! Bacteria are tougher little creatures than you might think, and dangerous varieties, such as listeria, thrive in colder temperatures. And these kinds of bacteria don't emit odors, so there's no way to know if they are present or not.

So, what to do? Here are some tips for keeping your fridge cleaner and safer.

- Keep your fridge and freezer cold. The refrigerator needs to be between 32°F and 40°F, while the freezer needs to be kept below 0°F to truly keep things frozen. Check the thermometer; if your fridge doesn't have one, buy two and keep them inside both areas. If things start to warm up, bacteria will grow. The danger zone for harmful bacteria is usually 40°F to 140°F.

- Don't put too much food and drink in there. It might seem like a great idea to stuff your fridge to capacity, but air needs to circulate to keep things cold. If there are too many food items inside, it can slow and decrease that circulation, and cause things to warm up, potentially leading to spoilage.

- Clean it out regularly. We like to joke about the mysterious alien life-forms growing in the back of the fridge, but that's not too far from the truth! Spills, residue, and anything left behind will encourage bacteria to grow. Cleaning once a week is ideal, and yes, that seems like a real chore! But once the hard work is done (because you've probably not cleaned it in, like, five years, right?), it will be easy enough to give the shelves and walls a quick rubdown. As usual, hot, soapy water or a one-part water to one-part vinegar mix will do just fine. Wear rubber gloves and with a sponge or cloth, be sure to get in to all the cracks and crevices. If your shelves are glass, a glass cleaner will also work.

- Clean the outside. Not just the handle, but the doors, the seals, everything.

- Studies have shown that the water and ice dispenser can be one of the most germ-infested areas of the fridge. Read your instruction manual on how to keep it clean.

- Pull out the whole unit and check behind it for debris and dust. Keep the motor and grill clear, so that dust doesn't collect and potentially damage the motor.

A little routine maintenance on your fridge will keep it running happily for years, and keep your food better protected!

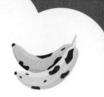

OLD FOOD *and* DRINK

Obviously, one of the biggest challenges to storing perishable food is keeping it fresh and consuming it before it goes off. It's not only a health issue, but spoiled food can make your fridge pretty stinky if it gets lost in the back somewhere and you forget about it . . . another reason not to overstuff your shelves!

Dangerous bacteria grow quite easily on spoiled food, the kinds that cause food poisoning and leave you hating life for a day or two and spending more time in your bathroom than you want to. And you won't always be able to tell if something is spoiled just by smelling it. So, follow these recommendations to keep your food safer.

- Don't store meat on the top shelves. Meat juices have a tendency to leak out and could seep down to lower shelves, contaminating other food. Also, since heat rises, it can actually be a bit warmer on the top shelf.

- Keep eggs in their original carton, not in the egg containers in the drawer. Studies have shown that this area can be too warm, and they may spoil sooner. Store them at the back of the fridge instead.

- Also, store milk in the refrigerator proper, not the door. It will keep cooler and last longer.

- Keep fruits and veggies separate, not together. Fruits emit a gas called ethylene that can increase the rate at which veggies spoil. So, if you have two crisper drawers, store them separately.

- Don't do things like pouring half a glass of milk back into a container! It's already been exposed to the air and other bacteria. Also, don't drink out of milk containers and put them back in the fridge. Pour what you need into a glass and keep the container fresh.

- Butter is surprisingly robust and can last one to three months in the refrigerator, whether it's been opened or not. Salted butter may last a bit longer than unsalted. Still, you should store it well, because it can absorb odors and flavors from surrounding foods which, if not dangerous, are unappetizing! You may wish to store it in a dedicated glass butter dish for extra protection. You can also freeze it for up to one year.

- Be careful with leftover rice. After it's been cooked, don't let it sit out for more than an hour. Refrigerate it as soon is it's cooled down enough to do so. Uncooked rice sometimes has spores of *bacillus cereus*, a kind of bacteria that causes food poisoning. It can survive at high temperatures, even after being cooked, so if the rice is left out after cooking at room temperature, the bacteria can begin to multiply. Refrigerating will stop this from happening, but be sure to eat up the remainder of the rice soon, preferably within a day. Also, don't reheat it more than once.

Food storage is a big subject, more than can be covered here, but taking some basic precautions will help your food last longer and keep you safer.

THE STOVE

Everything happens on the stove: food gets cooked, and it also spills over, leaving splotches and traces of things everywhere. It's easy to let these go for too long until you have a stove that's massively dirty and covered in food bits.

- A dirty stove looks gross, it's hard to clean, and it may harbor all kinds of bacteria. Just because the stove can get very hot doesn't mean that it will kill anything nearby.

- The stove handles will pick up whatever you've had on your hands, every time you turn them on and off. Have you been handling raw meat? Juices and the bacteria in them will happily slide off your fingers and onto the surface of the handle.

- Stove handles are often considered by some studies to be one of the most contaminated places in your kitchen!

Clearly, you need to make a commitment to keeping your stove clean. Here's how.

- Just tell yourself that you need to clean the stove. Go on! No matter what kind you have: gas or electric, the surface will get stained and splattered, and the more often you keep those stains from building up, the easier it will be to keep clean. A little bit every day or every other day will prevent the big job that you'll avoid and will only get worse.

- If you are fortunate enough to have a glass-top stove, these are easily cleaned, and you should wipe it down after every use with a glass cleaner or an all-purpose surface cleaner.

- If possible, periodically remove and clean the burners (electric) or the grill above the flame (gas). Check your manual for instructions if you are unsure how to remove them. Despite the heat they are subjected to, grit and residue will build up on them over time.

- Obviously, you can't wipe down the stove handles when you're in the middle of making a meal but be aware that they should be wiped down daily to ensure that no bacteria take hold. An equal part vinegar/hot water solution will do the trick for a daily rub and clean them with a commercial all-purpose cleaner or a dedicated oven cleaner once a week or so.

- For a deeper stove handle clean: the handles should be removable, so take them off and immerse them in hot, soapy water once every two weeks. Let them really soak, then rinse them off and let them dry completely before putting them back on.

The stove is the place you will prepare many, if not most, of your meals, so take the time to keep it clean and safe by doing a little every day.

THE KITCHEN VENT *and* RANGE HOOD

With daily use of the stove, range hoods can get dirty quickly, and it's usually a gross combination of dust and grease that gets stuck on! If you let it go for too long, it might seem impossible, thus leading you to put it off even longer. Then, it just gets even grosser!

As you can probably imagine, it's not just dirt that gets trapped under that grease. Germs, bacteria, mold, and all sort of things can take up residence in a place that's literally right in front of your face while you're cooking, so it's a good idea to get it clean and keep it clean. Fortunately, it's not that difficult.

- Cover your stove in plastic or a drop cloth; if you haven't cleaned the vent in a while, bits will probably start falling off as you do!

- First, you'll want to clean the outside. To cut through that grease, a good liquid dish soap will usually do the trick. Mix a bit in with some hot water to get it good and soapy, and then use a sponge or cloth to really get in there and get that grease off.

- Follow this clean with a spray of vinegar and water or a commercial surface cleaner, to get any remaining residue off.

- Clean the inside. If you've not done it in a while, this could be a real mess! A cloth or sponge might not be enough to get all the grime off. You might need to start with a gentle scrubbing brush to remove anything excessive and then switch to the soap-and-water method that you used to clean the outside.

- If something is really stuck on, mix a spoonful of baking soda with just enough water to form a paste, and spread it over the area. Wait for thirty minutes and then try cleaning again. The baking soda should help loosen up the sticky grit, so you can scrub it off.

- Clean the filter(s). This is just as important as cleaning the rest of the hood. If it's especially grimy and gross, wear gloves. Remove it according to the instructions. Fill your sink or another container with hot water and add a teaspoon of dishwashing liquid. Let the filter soak for fifteen to twenty minutes. Scrub it clean with a gentle brush but be careful not to damage the filter. Rinse and let it dry completely before replacing. Do this at least once a month.

- When the filter is out, check the vent itself for dirt and blockages. If you notice anything severe, you may need to consult a professional to have it cleaned.

Once you've done the odious task of getting all the grime off the range hood, it will be a snap to keep it clean, if you do light rubdown once a week or so, as part of your usual kitchen cleaning. This will keep away grime, germs, and debris.

THE OVEN

Like the stove, the oven is a central part of your culinary masterpieces. Or, at least it's a place to heat things up. And that heat will usually do a good job of killing off germs and bugs. But there are other problems, if you let the oven go too long without a good cleaning.

- If you let grease and grime build up, over time it can interfere with the flow of hot air. This can mean that parts of your food don't cook properly. And if foods are undercooked, that can mean bacteria survive and can make their way into your system as you eat.

- Excess grease can cause your oven to smoke, which can be dangerous all on its own. At the very least, it can make your food taste off.

- The smoke from these grease fires can release dangerous chemicals, such as carbon monoxide, sulphur dioxide, and nitrogen oxide, which you definitely don't want to be breathing.

So, what to do? Clean the oven, of course!

- Some ovens have self-cleaning options. These may sound great, but they honestly don't clean everything up, much as we might wish they did. This is a high heat setting that allows for incinerating leftover food bits. It can take hours to do, and then you still have to clean. Is it worth it? A lot of people think not, especially if you just keep your oven clean, anyway.

- Clean your oven regularly, at least once week.

- Remove the oven racks and let them soak in soapy hot water. Scrub off any remaining dirt and let them dry completely.

- Cleaning an oven is not that difficult. Water and white vinegar or baking soda will do the trick. Mix baking soda with enough water to form a paste, and then spread the paste around the inside of the oven, but not the parts that heat up! Leave it for several hours or overnight, and then use a damp cloth to wipe it away, and the grease with it. You may still need to scrape off any remaining stubborn stains.

- Spray the inside of the oven with a solution made of one part water to one part white vinegar. Wipe with a clean cloth to remove any remaining grit and grease.

- Always cook to a minimum food temperate of 165°F. Use a food thermometer in the thickest part of the food to check. This is the baseline over which bacteria are killed. Since so many recipes call for high oven temperatures, food should heat to this level pretty easily, and you should be fine. But again, make sure your oven is clean to allow for even heating.

- Once a week, wipe down the oven handles and controls with disinfectant and a cloth, or use commercial wipes.

While not a major haven for germs, keeping your oven clean is still essential to stop them from spreading.

THE MICROWAVE

Microwaves are amazingly convenient for everything from warming up leftovers to when we can't be bothered to cook anything from scratch. They've become as much a part of our lives as TVs and computers. But they come with some hazards; not radiation, but, you guessed it, germs and bacteria!

- Here's the thing: microwaves don't automatically kill bacteria in food. They provide heat, which does kill bacteria, but as we all know, microwaves don't always heat, things up evenly, even with a rotating microwave tray. We've all taken foods out that have been blistering hot in one place, and lukewarm in another. And those uncooked places may have lingering bacteria.

- In most cases, this uneven heating isn't a problem, as long as you cook the food for the required time. Everything will catch up, eventually.

- A bigger problem is the inside of the microwave itself. People assume that the radiation must kill bacteria on the insides or the tray, but this just isn't true. Studies have shown that bacteria like E. coli and salmonella can both live happily inside a microwave, even one that is used regularly!

So, how can you keep your microwave and your food safe? How can you ensure that your supply of quick and easy meals doesn't get interrupted? There's binge-watching to do, after all!

- Always follow the heating instructions for your food. If you do, and the food still seems to need more time, give it a little more, say, thirty-second increments, until it is hot all the way through.

- Defrost any frozen foods before reheating. This will help them heat up more evenly.

- Keep foods sealed in microwave-safe containers (i.e., ones that won't be damaged or catch fire) when heating, preferably on a microwave-safe plate that sits on top of the rotating platter.

- Clean your microwave; this should go without saying. Do it several times a week, inside and out; the door handle and buttons are also breeding grounds for whatever bacteria you may take into the kitchen on your hands. An all-purpose commercial cleaner should do the trick. In between cleanings, keep the handles and outside clean with disinfectant wipes.

The microwave is essential to modern life. But make sure that nonessential bacteria don't hitch a ride into your system when all you're trying to do is enjoy a day in front of the TV!

CUTTING BOARDS

Cutting boards are essential for working on any serious recipe. You likely have one or more, and if you only have one, you should get more. Many people ask which is best, wood or plastic? The honest answer is that both have advantages and drawbacks, and if kept clean, both will work well. A third option, bamboo, is becoming increasingly popular, since bamboo grows amazingly quickly and is an easily renewable resource. Whatever type you have, keeping them clean is essential.

- If you use the same cutting board for every food item, you are potentially cross-contaminating your whole meal. If you chop raw chicken on the board, and then only rinse it off before chopping up a tomato to add to your salad, you've just picked up all kinds of chicken bacteria and spread it to your fresh food!

- Over time, your knives will make slices and grooves in your board. Cracks in boards (regardless of type) can contain countless bacteria. One study showed that a typical cutting board can have 200 percent more fecal bacteria than a toilet seat!

- Without a thorough cleaning after each use, those bacteria will only multiply and be waiting for your next chopping job . . . .

- So, cleaning your boards is essential. Here's how.

- Whatever kind of material you choose, keep dedicated cutting boards for different food items (meat, vegetables, other items, etc.) and don't mix them up, even after they've been washed.

- Wash plastic boards in your dishwasher after every use. This should be enough to keep them clean and sterilized.

- Wash wooden and bamboo boards with hot, soapy water and a good sponge or cloth.

- Every few weeks, soak your wooden and bamboo boards in a solution of one tablespoon of bleach mixed into a gallon of warm water. Let them sit for a few minutes, before removing and washing completely.

- Discard old boards when they get too cut up. Bacteria like E. coli and salmonella can build up in them over time, even if you keep them clean.

Cutting boards can be a primary place where germs are transmitted to and from food, but you can head them off at the pass with a little bit of extra care and preparation.

KNIVES *and* KNIFE BLOCKS

Knives are essential kitchen tools, but they can spread germs, if you're not careful. This is done either by contamination, or not keeping the knife block (or other storage) clean enough.

- If you store knives in a drawer, even if they are clean, they can pick up contaminants from their storage area, if it's not cleaned regularly.

- If you have a wooden knife block, bacteria can grow in the thin and dark crevices where you insert the knives, even if those knives are clean and spotless. Bet you never even thought of that!

- It goes without saying that if you don't clean your knives properly after each use, bacteria can multiply and potentially be risky later on.

So what's to be done to keep your knives cleaner and safer?

- If you use a knife for cutting meat, never reuse it for anything else until you've washed it thoroughly. If possible, have knives dedicated to certain foods, and don't use them in other contexts.

- This is really true for cutting any foods; don't just start a new cutting job, wash the knife off with soap and water before each reuse.

- If you keep your knives in a container, clean that container regularly with dish washing liquid and hot water. You can further soak it or wipe it down with a one-part vinegar and one-part water solution. Let it dry thoroughly before replacing it in a drawer or wherever you have it.

- If you just put your knives in a drawer, empty it out and clean it with a vinegar and water solution, using a cloth and a toothbrush to get into crevices. You'll be surprised at how much dirt you get out of a drawer, even when you keep it closed most of the time!

- If you have a knife block, wash it in hot and soapy water. Then, sterilize it by mixing a tablespoon of bleach into a gallon of warm water. Immerse the block in the water if you can; otherwise, pour some of the water/bleach mix into each knife slot. In either case, wait about a minute and then drain the block, and wash thoroughly again. Turn it over to let the water drain from the slots and leave until the block is completely dry. Do this at least once a month.

Keeping your knives cleaner will go a long way to keeping foods like meats and dairy safer.

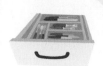

CUTLERY *and* CUTLERY DRAWERS

We use plates, cups, and cutlery every day, and they are essential to our meals, unless you're ordering out or eating only on paper plates. In most cases, giving them a good hot wash and dry in a dishwasher will be enough to keep them clean and germ-free. If you hand-wash, a good dose of liquid detergent and hot water should also be enough to get rid of whatever might be hanging out on that knife or fork, but there's probably one area you haven't thought of: the cutlery drawer!

- The place where you store your knives and forks is actually a breeding ground for germs, like so many other hidden corners and crevices of your kitchen.

- One study showed that the average cutlery container in a drawer had about as much bacteria as a toilet seat, and four times as much as a toilet handle.

- This is also true if you're just throwing your spoons, forks, and knives into a drawer without organizing them. It might even be worse in that case.

- If someone is reaching in there to get a random spoon or fork and hasn't washed their hands properly, it's just going to transfer those germs to your nice clean cutlery. And to the container holding them.

So, even after you wash your cutlery to a squeaky-clean state, you may be setting them down into a germ-infested storage area! Here's how to not do that.

- Keep the drawer clean! If you have a container in the drawer, take it out at least once a week and wash it with soap and hot water. Plastic containers are easy to clean, while a wooden container might prove a bit trickier (it can't go in your dishwasher, for example!). Give it a rub down with a damp cloth and clean with some disinfectant wipes. Be sure to let it dry completely before replacing it in the drawer.

- Periodically sanitize the container with one part white vinegar mixed into one part water. For a plastic container, you can pour this mixture in and let it sit. For a wooden one, you may want to use a cloth and go over the surfaces by hand.

- Use a toothbrush to get into any cracks and crevices in the container; get that vinegar solution ground in!

- Make sure the container is completely dry before returning utensils to it.

- If you're just throwing utensils into a drawer, remove them and clean it out with a water/vinegar solution, and then consider getting a simple container to hold your cutlery. It will be much easier to keep clean.

The cutlery drawer is often forgotten about, but it can ruin all of your hard work to keep your utensils clean, so don't neglect it!

STORAGE CONTAINERS

Plastic and glass containers are great for keeping leftovers, but there are usually two problems: people put food in containers that can end up getting shoved to the back of the fridge to be forgotten until said food looks like something out of a horror movie; and even when food is used up and the containers washed, there can be lingering food particles in the lids and seals where bacteria can thrive and multiply.

- A recent study of these lids found traces of salmonella and mold, as well as yeast, all of which you could be ingesting if you use the container again without storing it properly.

- Plastic containers can also hold onto smells and stains from previous foods, and these can leach into the food you want to store now. This is especially true of tomato-based foods, and those with mustard, turmeric, etc.

- Even if you use glass, the lids are usually plastic or rubber, so the problem can be there.

Fortunately, it's simple to keep your containers clean and germ-free.

- For lingering odors, stir four tablespoons of baking soda into a quart of warm water. If the container is small, immerse it in the water, if it won't fit, pour the water into the container itself. Let it soak for thirty minutes and then wash with soap and water. This removes unpleasant odors and gives your containers a fresher look and feel.

- For stains, add a tablespoon of liquid chlorine bleach to a cup of warm water, and pour into the container. Add one tablespoon for each additional cup of water you need to cover the stain. Let it sit for thirty minutes and then wash thoroughly in hot water and soap. Be sure to rinse out any remaining traces of bleach before using again.

- Wash containers and lids in the top shelf of your dishwasher, if you have one. If not, use a good liquid detergent and make sure to really scrub the lids and seals. Dry them well; you can put them in direct sunlight to dry off, which will help kill harmful bacteria.

- Never let a container live for months in your fridge. You're just asking for bacterial trouble, along with bad smells and a potential horror show of unknown final growths and other surprises!

Containers are great for keeping extra food on hand. Just be smart about keeping them clean and safe to use.

BLENDERS *and* OTHER TOOLS

You may have all kinds of handy appliances in your kitchen: a blender and/or food processor, an electric can opener, a coffee maker, and so on. But do these appliances contain potentially harmful bacteria? Of course they do!

- Studies of appliances have found that over 25 percent of them carry such nasties as E. coli and salmonella, 10 percent had listeria, and virtually all of them had some kind of mold.

- Blenders are particularly bad for mold.

- Blenders, coffee makers, and can openers are among the most germ-infested of all the objects that the study team tested.

Yikes! But fear not, as with everything in the kitchen, keeping your appliances clean is the first and best way to reduce germs.

- A manual can opener can be washed in the dishwasher or soaked in hot soapy water. As usual, a one part white vinegar to one-part water solution can be great to soak in and disinfect. Electric can openers can be more difficult to clean, and some parts might be inaccessible. Consult your manual for advice on how to clean it, so as not to damage any interior electronic parts.

- Rinse your blender or food processor blades after each use, to prevent food from getting stuck on and built up. If the blades are removable, do so with care, and soak in warm, soapy water. Be wary of putting these parts in a dishwasher, even if the manual says it's safe to do so; the hot water and harsh detergents can damage blades over time. Don't use abrasive cleaners or harsh scrubbing pads, as these can also damage the blades.

- You can also clean your blender by filling it about halfway with warm water and adding a few drops of liquid dish soap. Put the lid on and run on the lowest setting to let the inside get a good wash. Rinse after with warm water.

- Clean your drip-style coffee maker at least once a month (more if you use it heavily) by filling the reservoir with a blend of one part white distilled vinegar and one part water. Put a filter in the basket and turn the machine on. When it's about half finished, turn the machine off; the water and vinegar that are left over will slowly seep through (this may take up to an hour). Turn the machine back on to finish. Follow this with two more washes of plain water to flush out any remaining vinegar smell, and your coffee maker will be clean, disinfected, and ready to use.

Simple appliances don't have to cause big headaches when you're cleaning. But it's worth taking the time to keep them clean, so add them to your weekly cleaning routines.

THE DISHWASHER

You might think that the dishwasher, with its concentrated detergent and hot blasting water, would be the one place where germs can't possibly survive. And you'd be wrong. Given the extreme conditions of a dishwasher (hot to cold, wet to dry), it can be a place where all sorts of little things take up residence, especially on the rubber seals.

- One study found bacteria such as pseudomonas, Escherichia, and acinetobacter thriving. The good news is that these are common and mostly harmless, though some strains can cause problems for people with compromised immune systems.

- The study also found fungi such as candida and cryptococcus, which can cause opportunistic and fungal infections.

- Fungi usually come from the water that circulates through the machine, while bacteria probably come from food.

- Generally, these bacteria and mold are not harmful, unless someone is immunocompromised, but it's still a good idea to keep the appliance as clean as possible.

- Remove the racks and wash and scrub in hot soapy water at least once a month.

- Check the drain and sides for food residue and buildup. A paste of baking soda and water, left on for fifteen minutes, should be enough to remove anything that's stuck on.

- For a simple way to disinfect your dishwasher, fill a dishwasher-safe container with one cup of white vinegar and set it upright in the upper rack of the machine. Put nothing else in and run the dishwasher on a normal cleaning cycle with hot water. This will spread around the vinegar and easily clean and disinfect inside. Do this once a month.

- For a stronger clean, you can fill the dishwasher detergent compartment with powdered laundry bleach and run (again empty) on a hot water setting. As with the vinegar cleaning, try this once a month for a deeper clean. A commercial cleaner, such as Affresh Washer Cleaner, is also effective.

- Apply disinfectant to the rubber seal, and clean with a sponge or cloth. Use a toothbrush to scrub into crevices. You can also use a solution of one part bleach to nine parts water, which is good for scrubbing out the entire inside of the machine.

Dishwashers probably present little danger of transmitting harmful bacteria or mold, but it's better to be safe than sorry, so a periodic clean-out of the machine will ensure that it stays safe and continues working optimally.

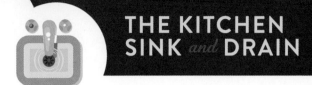

THE KITCHEN
SINK *and* DRAIN

Bad news: the kitchen sink is practically a convention center for germs. Just how many?

- A study by the Global Hygiene Council found that kitchen sinks have over 17,000 bacteria per square inch, and 13,000 bacteria per square inch on and around the handles of the tap (see the next section for cleaning those handles).

- Many of these bacteria were harmless, but E. coli and salmonella were also present.

- Another study found that nearly half of all sinks had coliform bacteria, and over a quarter of them had mold.

- In Britain, the National Health Service found that kitchen sinks can contain up to 100,000 times more germs than a bathroom! And this is one of the most important places for preparing your food!

Clearly, keeping the kitchen sink and drain as clean as possible is essential.

- If you drop a bit of food into your sink, just let it go. There's no "five second rule" for kitchen sinks! Or anywhere, for that matter.

- Clean your sink at least once a week with a good disinfectant. Spray it on and scrub.

- Sometimes, you'll want to do a deeper clean to remove stains. For porcelain sinks, sprinkle baking soda to coat the sink, then drizzle a few drops of hydrogen peroxide into the sink and scrub with a sponge or brush. This will remove stains and keep it glowing white!

- For a deeper clean for stainless steel sinks: again, use baking soda, but instead of hydrogen peroxide, add a bit of dish soap and scrub.

- To clean your drain in an environmentally friendly way, take one part baking soda and two parts white vinegar. Sprinkle the soda down the drain, and then slowly pour the white vinegar in. Yes, this will cause a reaction and it will bubble (remember those volcano science projects as a kid?), but that's the point! Leave for fifteen minutes and then flush hot water down the drain. This will not only kill germs and stop odors, but also it's a great way to clear blockages. And make a mini volcano!

- If you have a grate or plug hole over your drain, it's essential to clean it regularly, since it's practically an invitation to bacteria to set up camp! Empty any debris caught in it, and use a toothbrush or other small brush to remove the gunk and buildup. Wash it thoroughly with hot water and soap (or run it through the dishwasher, if it's safe to so), and disinfect with a spray. Do this every two to three days to ensure that it stays (mostly) germ-free and stays clear to allow water to drain properly.

Cleaning the sink takes a bit more attention, but it's an essential part of your daily food-prep routine, so you need to look after it.

THE KITCHEN FAUCET

This is probably not a surprise, but the kitchen faucet and its handles can be one of the germier places in your kitchen. You go to wash your hands to get rid of germs, but as soon as you touch the handles to start the flow of water, you transfer germs to the handle(s). Then, when you go to turn the faucet off, those germs jump right back on your clean hands! It's a vicious circle from which you cannot escape! Or can you?

- Whatever germs are on your hands will transfer to the faucet handles and the tap, just waiting to jump on to whoever uses them next.

- Studies have found all kinds of bacteria lurking on those handles, including staphylococcus, as well as mold and other growing things.

- Over time, the faucet itself will get overgrown with bacteria, mold, lime scale, and mildew, all of which can hitch a ride into your water. At the very least, it can ruin the taste of your refreshing drink!

Cleaning the faucet is easy but shouldn't be neglected.

- Do a daily wipe-down of the handles and all of the hardware with wipes or a spray-on disinfectant and a cloth. This won't take long and will drastically reduce buildup and bacteria of any kind. It will make it safer for you when you're in the kitchen and handling food.

- For cleaning the faucet itself, there's an easy way to remove buildup where the water comes out. Fill a small plastic bag about halfway with white vinegar. Put the bag over the nozzle to cover the opening, and immerse it in the vinegar. Secure to the faucet with a rubber band or elastic tie. Let it soak for half an hour or so.

- Remove the bag and discard the vinegar. It will have done a wonderful job of removing buildups and killing germs. Now get in there with a gentle brush and remove anything remaining. Rinse with warm water and it will be clean! Do this once a week or so, and you'll never have to worry about mold or mildew again, as well as keeping the germ population way down!

Keeping the kitchen faucet clean is easy and is a first point of defense to protect that most precious resource that we need every day.

DISH TOWELS

Even if you have a dishwasher, you probably have a few towels hanging up in your kitchen to do quick drying for things you need right away. You may also use them to mop up spills and other mini disasters. And guess what? They're probably full of bacteria!

- Studies have shown that a large number of towels (more than half in one case) were contaminated with bacteria like E. coli, and staphylococcus.

- Towels that get wet and are used and reused without being able to dry out are a big culprit in bacterial growth. This is especially true in areas that are more humid.

- Towel that are used for multiple purposes usually have much higher counts of bacteria, since they can pick them up from many locations.

- If you're using damp dish towels and then going to prepare food without washing your hands, you're just spreading all those germs right to your food.

Yuck! Fortunately, keeping your towels safe isn't a difficult task.

- Wash your hands frequently. As always, this lowers the risk of transferring germs from once surface to another. Always wash before preparing food or using your towels.

- Keep separate towels for separate duties. Have one or two for cleaning up stains, and another only for drying off dishes or utensils that you're using. Don't let them cross over.

- Wash the towels for stains and spills every day or every other day, in hot water. Wash your drying towels at least once a week, also in hot water. If they're color-safe, consider adding bleach to the wash.

- Dry them in your dryer, if you have one. This will finish the job of killing harmful bacteria.

- Try to keep towels in an area of the kitchen where they will dry out and not stay damp between uses. This slows down the growth of bacteria. Let them hang freely from a rack or bar; don't fold them up and stack them after using.

- Consider using paper towels for some jobs, such as wiping up spills. While cloth towels are more environmentally sound, in some cases, it might be better to use paper ones that you can just throw away.

Keeping your towels clean needs to be one of your daily kitchen jobs; just make it a part of your normal laundering to clean towels thoroughly.

THE PANTRY

The pantry is a crucial place for storing foods of all kinds, mainly of the dry and canned varieties, so it should be pretty safe from germs, right? Think again. The problem is that things like rice, pasta, etc. can leak out if not sealed properly, and attract insects and vermin.

- If your dry food is not properly sealed, it can let in moisture which can lead to mold and yeast growth in the food itself. This is especially true if you leave some bags and containers for a long time without checking them.

- Food that's improperly stored will easily attract visitors. You know how ants love a picnic? Well, if there's an ongoing picnic in your pantry, guess who's going to show up?

- If your pantry is attracting mice or other small creatures, they will leave droppings, which can have all sorts of bacteria in them.

Cleaning the pantry doesn't have to be a big chore if you follow these tips regularly.

- Always store rice, pasta, beans, and other dried goods in well-sealed containers, preferably glass jars. Don't use plastic bags, or just leave them in the store bags they came in. This will keep them fresher for longer and reduce the risk of leakage and vermin attraction.

- Make it a routine to remove all the jars and containers once a month or so, and wipe them down to remove dust and grit that may have accumulated.

- Discard anything that has expired. That can of soup that was "best by" July 2003? Yeah, chuck it out!

- While the containers are out, clean your pantry shelves. Use a paper towel or clean cloth to wipe off any bigger bits or grit, and then dust them to remove regular dust. Wipe clean with a damp cloth and use an all-purpose surface cleaner. Let them dry completely before putting back containers.

- Look for any signs of animal droppings, chew marks, insects (especially ants), and so on. If you're keeping the shelves clean regularly, you probably won't have a problem, but check often just to be sure. If you see evidence of animal droppings, look for a source where the animal may be entering. You may need to consult a professional for this if you have an infestation.

- When putting things back, it's a good idea to organize them by type: rice in one area, pasta in another, etc. This makes it less likely that one container or can will get hidden behind another container and not used for months, or years!

- When you use up the contents of a container, run it through the dishwasher or give it a good hand-wash in hot soapy water. Be sure to let it dry completely before refilling.

Keeping a clean pantry will keep your dry goods healthier and fresher, and prevent unwanted visitors of all sizes, from microorganisms to mice.

CLEANING SPONGES

So, you may have heard the deal with kitchen sponges. They are magnets for germs and bacteria of just about every kind.

- A kitchen sponge can contain concentrations of bacteria as high as the human intestinal tract.

- Another study found over 360 types of bacteria on one set of kitchen sponges! And five of the ten most commonly found bacteria on these had "pathogenic potential."

- While many of these bacteria are harmless, the kinds you don't want can easily take root and grow, especially if you've been cleaning dishes or spills from food that's prone to harboring them.

- As you're probably not surprised to learn, your kitchen sponge often has more bacteria than your toilet—the same sponge you use to clean your plates and such.

How do you keep these germ factories from getting out of hand? By keeping them clean, designating tasks, and getting rid of them frequently! Here's what to do.

- Wash your hands before handling any sponge. Wash them again afterward.

- Keep different sponges for different purposes. Never use a dish sponge to clean up the countertops, much less the sink. Have dedicated sponges for different tasks: one (or more) for dishes, one for countertops, one for wiping down handles and knobs, etc. Use different colors for each sponge, or snip off the corner of one to identify them.

- Rinse a sponge out with extra soap after each use and set it aside to dry.

- Let your sponges dry out completely between uses. Don't stack them in places where they will retain moisture. A rack is the best option. Don't just leave them on the countertop.

- Some sponges can be cleaned, both in the microwave and the washing machine (with hot water). Be careful when microwaving, though. Sponges that are synthetic or have metal fibers can catch fire in microwaves. Be sure to microwave sponges when they are still wet (soak it in water if you need to), since the steam from heating helps to kill germs. Microwaving a dry sponge could also cause a fire. Set the microwave to high and run for two minutes.

- Rotate your sponges out regularly and discard used ones. Don't let them get too worn and tattered. Some experts recommend that you change them out once a week, if you do a lot of washing; certainly, you shouldn't be keeping them for months at a time!

Sponges are a necessary tool in the kitchen, so use them wisely, and you'll cut down on the huge number of bacteria they can breed.

GARBAGE DISPOSALS

Like drains, garbage disposals come into contact with just about every germ imaginable. And since they process old food, egg shells, discarded meat parts, etc., it means that bits and particles get stuck in them. Over time, bacteria will grow spectacularly well, which can be dangerous, bad-smelling, or both. Since we've already seen that a sink can have a half million bacteria or more, imagine what's going on in the disposal!

- Whatever germs are in there will be a combination of whatever was on the food you put down it, and other general germs and bacteria that grow in damp places.

- The disposal can develop a nasty slime on it over time if it's not kept clean, which can produce unpleasant odors.

Here's how to keep your disposal much cleaner and (relatively) germ-free.

- Dump a tray of ice cubes into the disposal, topped off by a half cup of salt. Run a thin stream of water from the faucet into the disposal. Turn it on and with a long, wooden spoon (or something similar), gently push all the ice and salt into the disposal. Let run for a minute or two, and then turn the water off.

- Pour half a cup of backing soda into the disposal followed by one cup of white vinegar. Yes, it will fizzle and bubble. This is good. Let this volcanic mixture sit for fifteen to twenty minutes, before flushing with hot water.

- You may need to get in deeper with a scrub brush. If so, turn off the fuse or power source for the disposal. Always! Don't take any chances. We've probably all seen one gross-out horror movie or another where someone doesn't do this, and the results are disastrous.

- If your disposal has a removable splash guard, take it off now, and soak it in an equal water/vinegar or nine-parts water/one-part bleach solution for several minutes. Wash completely with soap and water and let it dry.

- For long-term maintenance, don't pour used grease and oil down the disposal or your drain. Over time, this will gum up the mechanism and make it work less efficiently.

If you have a garbage disposal, it's essential to keep it clean, but with a little regular maintenance, it shouldn't give you any problems.

FRUIT BOWLS *and* VEGGIE BASKETS

It's nice to be able to have fresh fruit on hand, to pick up a piece from your fruit bowl, rinse it off, and dig in, but as you're probably already guessing, fruit and veggie bowls can be bad news. How bad? One study showed that the average fruit bowl was over 160 times dirtier than just throwing your fruit in the kitchen sink and leaving it there. Wow!

- Fruit ripens and then rots. How often have you pulled a piece of fruit or a vegetable out of the bowl, one that's been sitting on the bottom, only to find it's rotting away, gone moldy, has white fuzz all over it, etc.? It's not only annoying, but also it's leaving behind countless bacteria in your bowl.

- If you haven't washed your hands properly, putting your hands into the bowl is going to spread around germs. Even if you thoroughly wash the piece of fruit you've taken (and you should!), the germs remain behind in the bowl.

- If you don't clean your fruit bowl regularly, bacteria and germs will just sit in there and multiply. The organic, moist environment of a piece of fruit or vegetable is ideal for microscopic things to come out and party.

With a little extra fruit bowl knowledge, you can prevent unpleasant surprises at the bottom.

- Wash your hands before putting them into the bowl to retrieve anything.

- Wash the fruit or vegetables thoroughly to wash away any germs that have accumulated while they were in the bowl.

- Make an effort to use up your fresh produce regularly. Most of it won't keep long; if you bought it, eat it!

- Minimize fruit rot by storing things strategically: apples do better in the fridge, while bananas should not be stored there. Citrus fruits do fine at room temperature, while berries of all kinds need to be refrigerated. For refrigerated fruits and veggies, store them in the crisper drawers, with fruits in one and veggies in the other.

- Wash your fruit bowls or containers regularly in hot soapy water or put them in the dishwasher if they are dishwasher-safe. Do this every time before you restock them.

It's not difficult to stop germs and bacteria from getting out of hand in your produce bowls. Just clean them, eat all your fruits and veggies, and you'll be fine!

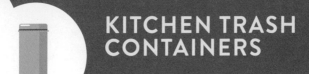

KITCHEN TRASH CONTAINERS

So, we've saved the worst for last. As you can probably imagine, the kitchen trash can has the potential to be one of the worst offenders of all when it comes to harboring and spreading germs, since all of your outcast stuff goes in it. It's a place where germs go to party, socialize, multiply, and thrive, and you can't do anything about it, or can you?

- Depending on what you're throwing out, salmonella, E. coli, and listeria can all thrive in your bin.

- The longer you leave things rotting away in your trash bin, the more bacteria will grow, including odor-causing ones that can stink up your whole kitchen, even your whole home. We've all walked into our kitchens and noticed a funky smell at one time or another. Usually it's only then that we're reminded that it's time to take out the trash.

Fortunately, it's pretty easy enough to prevent dirt and germs from taking over. Do these things to keep your bin clean and odor-free.

- Always use plastic bag bin liners that are dedicated for trash bins. The reason is obvious, since you can just lift the bag and its contents out and throw it away. If you're just tossing things into a plastic bin, it's going to get real gross, real fast, and you'll have a lot more cleaning to do!

- Once the plastic bag is out, it's time to clean the bin itself. This can be done with a simple hot water and dish soap mix and some scrubbing. Or if you want to disinfect it more and get rid of any lingering trash odors, add three-quarters cup of bleach to a gallon of hot water. Pour this mix into the bin and let it sit for at least fifteen minutes.

- You can also use white vinegar or an equal water/vinegar mix, but **never mix bleach with vinegar or bleach with ammonia!** This will release a toxic gas that can be dangerous, even deadly. When cleaning your bin, choose one of these and mix it with water only.

- Wash the bin thoroughly and rinse out. Turn it over to let the excess water drain out. This is obviously best done outside!

- Let the bin air-dry completely before putting a new bin liner in.

- Do this cleaning after each time you take the plastic bag out to the outside trash.

The kitchen trash bin might seem like a place of horror, and it can be, but keeping germs contained in a bag and doing a regular cleaning will keep it from becoming monstrous!

CHAPTER 3:

GERMS IN THE BATHROOM

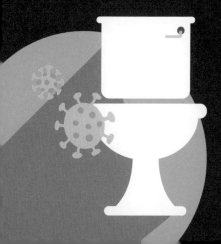

You might be thinking that the bathroom is the most likely place in the house for germs and bacteria to show up, and that they'll be at their worst there. Well, depending on the home, this may be true! At the very least, it's probably tied with your kitchen. We already associate the bathroom with germs and uncleanliness in general, simply because the toilet is there, and it's the room we use to scrub off the day's dirt. And it's true, these two things can be prime sources of bacteria. So, it's essential to keep the bathroom extra clean and shiny to keep the spread of germs down.

This chapter will uncover all the unpleasantness of your germ-infested bathroom: places you might have suspected needed a bit more cleaning, and some that you've probably never thought of. Keeping the bathroom clean might take a bit of extra effort, but it's not difficult and will go a long way to controlling the spread of germs, viruses, and bacteria in the area where you're trying to be rid of them.

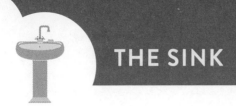

THE SINK

Yes, it's true: your bathroom sink and drain, just like your kitchen sink, is an absolute haven for germs. Thankfully, you're not preparing food in your bathroom (or . . . are you?), so that's one concern removed. But that doesn't mean that your sink is all fine. You'll probably be distressed to learn a few facts.

- Studies have shown that the bathroom sink can be even more contaminated than the toilet.

- Think about everything you put down it just in the course of getting ready to go somewhere: bacteria from washing your hands after using the toilet, spit from toothpaste, skin detritus from razors, blood from razor cuts or toothpaste, and so on. Most of the bacteria will just wash away, but not all.

The good news is that keeping the sink clean is not difficult, and it's already a part of your bathroom cleaning routine.

- Keep doing what you're doing. Make sure to wipe down the handles and faucet with disinfectant wipes or a cleaning spray and a cloth. Do this more often than you're probably doing it; every other day would be good, or even every day, if the bathroom is used by several people.

- As with the kitchen sink, sprinkle baking soda to coat the sink bowl, and then drizzle a few drops of hydrogen peroxide into the sink and scrub with a sponge or brush. Hydrogen peroxide can be used safely in porcelain and stainless-steel sinks and will remove any built-up stains and keep it clean.

- Use the same method for cleaning the bathroom sink as for the kitchen sink: To clean your drain in an environmentally friendly way, take one part baking soda and two parts white vinegar. Sprinkle the soda down the drain, and then slowly pour the white vinegar in. Let it bubble and leave for at least fifteen minutes before pouring hot water down the drain. This will stop odors and unclog blockages. Use it regularly to keep your sink drain, well, draining.

- If you have a removable hair catcher or other screen over the drain, remove it and soak it in a one-part bleach to nine-parts water solution for five to ten minutes. Wash completely with hot water and soap before returning the stopper to the drain hole. Use a toothbrush to scrub out any particles trapped in the mesh.

Your bathroom sink is an essential part of getting ready in the morning and winding down in the evening. Just make sure to keep it clean as part of your normal cleaning routine. Adding these few extra touches will ensure that it's safe and clean for the whole family.

THE TOILET

As you're probably well aware, the toilet is a prime collector of germs and bacteria, and keeping it clean is essential. No doubt you already clean it pretty regularly. But do you know just what's lurking in the bowl and on the lid?

- Obviously, fecal bacteria go into your toilet bowl every day, so there's always a new supply, no matter how often you clean it. This is normal and to be expected. It just means that you'll need to clean the toilet more often that you probably do.

- Toilets are definitely infested with germs, but not as many as you might think; toothbrush holders actually have more (see below).

Fortunately, we tend to keep toilets cleaner already, since we perceive them as being dirty, germy environments. Here are some simple ways to keep your toilet as clean as possible.

- Always put the lid down before you flush. Flushing with the lid up can scatter an astonishing quantity of bacteria from feces and water drops. Hundreds, even thousands, of microbes per square inch can thrive in the toilet, so if you flush with the lid up, you're basically turning it into an aerosol that sprays back on you and the bathroom. Drops from toilet water can splash out as far as six to eight feet! Just make sure that you clean the inside of the lid regularly, since all of that bacteria-laden water is splashing up onto it.

- Keep your toilet bowl clean using whatever method you already do, such as a bristle scrubbing brush, commercial toilet bowl cleaner, and wipes for the sides, back, and handle. Always wear rubber gloves when cleaning a toilet. If you want to try something less harsh, toss one-half cup of baking soda and one-quarter cup of white vinegar into the bowl and let it bubble. Swish it around with a toilet brush and let it sit for at least twenty minutes (you can leave it for several hours, if possible). This will clean, disinfect, and control odor.

- Wipe down both sides of the seat and the lid with disinfectant and a cleaning cloth, as well as the outside of the bowl, the cover for the water basin, etc.

- Clean the flush handle daily with disinfectant wipes, since this will be touched by unwashed hands on a regular basis.

- Wash your hands, before and after using the toilet. Prevent the spread of bacteria by keeping them as clean as possible.

You already clean your toilet, so take a few extra steps to make sure it's as clean as it can be.

THE SHOWER

Nothing refreshes like a hot shower! But is your shower nozzle as clean as it should be? Probably not.

- A study of fifty showerheads from around the US revealed a shocking fact: almost one-third of them were infested with a type of bacteria known as mycobacterium avium, which can cause lung infections and disease when inhaled. This can cause dry cough, trouble breathing, and fatigue.

- When you turn the shower on and splash that hot water on your face and inhale the steam, you might well be getting a lungful of mycobacterium avium!

- Mold and yeast also live in wet showerheads.

- Bacteria can line the walls of showers and attach themselves to you.

Fortunately, you don't have to give up your showers! Just keep the head clean; here's how.

- Start cleaning your showerhead at least once a week. Unscrew it and give it a good clean. You might find a slimy residue on the inside, and that's where mycobacteria like to thrive, so get it cleaned out.

- Soaking in a one-part bleach to nine-parts water solution is good, while ammonia is also a good disinfectant for killing mycobacteria (just **never** mix ammonia and bleach!). After soaking, wash thoroughly with soap and water and rinse clean. Let the head dry out completely before reattaching it to the shower.

- A metal showerhead is not necessarily better or cleaner. Some studies have shown that these have as much, or even more, bacteria than their plastic counterparts.

- Scientists stress that you're not likely top pick up a mycobacterium infection from splashing water on your face, or even swallowing it, unless your immune system is suppressed, but it's better to be safe than sorry.

- Use an easy-to-clean, rust-free shower rack to store your shampoo bottles, soap, and such.

- Clean and wipe down the walls with vinegar or a commercial cleaner regularly, preferably after each time someone uses the shower. This will reduce bacteria and mold growth. Use a spray bottle and let sit for five to ten minutes. Wipe clean with a cloth or a squeegee.

- Spray your shower curtain with a water-vinegar *or* a water-bleach mix (one part water to one part vinegar, and one part bleach to ten parts water), to control mold and mildew. *Never* mix bleach and vinegar! After a shower, make sure to spread out the curtain to let it dry. Don't leave it bunched up to one side or the other.

- Don't let mold build up in your shower tiles. Use a commercial shower tile cleaner or a water-bleach spray to keep it under control.

- Keep your bathroom ventilated and prevent mist from lingering. A ceiling fan vent or open window will do the trick.

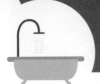

THE BATHTUB

There's nothing like taking a nice, hot bath to soak away your troubles. But if you're not cleaning your bathtub regularly, you're basically swimming in a bacteria soup!

- Studies have shown that there are up to 200,000 bacteria per square inch in an average bathtub.

- This includes those old favorites like E. coli, streptococcus, and staphylococcus.

- If you're getting into the tub with the dirt and grime of the day on you, it's going to float off of you but stay in the water. So you're floating in your own filth. Lovely.

- Since bathtubs can take a while to dry out, the bacteria will only multiply over time, and be ready to go for a swim as soon as you fill up the tub with nice, hot water again.

But fear not! You don't have to give up on bubble baths just yet! Here's what you can do to make your soak time cleaner and safer.

- Shower first. Wash off all the day's dirt *before* you take a bath. You'll be getting into the water clean and there's less chance of anything unpleasant floating off of you and into the water, only to hang around.

- Don't use the bath as a place to actually bathe. Scrubbing the dirt off you just leaves it in the water, where it can float around and stick to other places on your body.

- Keep the tub clean at all times, either with a commercial bathtub cleaner, or a mix of one part water to one part white vinegar. Give the tub a good scrubbing and watch out for cracks or mold growth. Keep the drain and the plug clean. Soak the plug in a solution of water and vinegar, or a one-part bleach to nine-parts water mix for at least fifteen minutes. Then scrub with hot, soapy water and let dry completely.

- If you can clean on the day you're going to have a bath, even better, but try to clean out the tub as part of your cleaning routine, once a week or more if you take baths frequently.

- If you have children, don't keep their bath toys in the tub; these can be prime breeding grounds for bacteria. Wash in the dishwasher if possible, and store them in a dry area, such as a bath net or a dedicated toy holder and drainer. Only bring them out when needed. Some parents recommend discarding any toys that can't be cleaned properly after three to six months. Use your judgment. Keep waterproof bath books clean by scrubbing them down after every bath.

Yes, you can still have your bubble baths and sip champagne in luxury, but just take some care to make sure that your bath is an enjoyable experience, not an invitation to germs!

YOUR RAZOR

If you use a straight razor to shave, you've probably already heard the drill: you need to swap them out pretty often. And there are good reasons for this.

- Your skin is naturally covered in bacteria (mostly harmless), but when you shave, you are scraping off layers of skin cells and bacteria that will remain on the blades.

- If you have a bacteria-infested razor, you won't know, but it can cause irritations like folliculitis (inflammation of the hair follicle). Then, you'll definitely know it!

- Yeast and mold can also grow on a razor and blades, since bathrooms tend to get hot and steamy.

- If you borrow a razor from someone else, you're increasing your chances of infection.

So, here's how to shave without the consequences.

- Use a one- or two-blade razor. Any more than that can damage your skin and leave you more susceptible to infections.

- If you shave daily, change your razors regularly, no more than every three to four days. Razors get duller with each use, meaning that you're more likely to cut yourself, since you'll have to press down harder to get the same close shave each time. If you cut yourself, you're leaving your body open to infection, not only from bacteria, but also other things like yeast and mold that may be on the blades. Your skin acts as a natural barrier to these, but only if it's unbroken.

- If you have any kind of skin condition or infection, either try not to shave near it or discard the blade after each use. Otherwise, you can pass the infection on to the blade and spread it around if you're shaving more than one area.

- Don't store your razor in the shower. After a shower, the leftover heat and steam are perfect for allowing bacteria and fungi to flourish on the blades. Rinse it out completely to remove any remaining hairs or shaving cream, dip in rubbing alcohol, and dry off with a paper towel. Store your razor in a cool, dry place.

- Don't share razors with a partner or friend. This drastically increases the chances of spreading infection, anything from staph infections to fungal growths on the skin. Even serious viruses, like hepatitis and herpes, can linger on a blade. Keep your blades to yourself!

Love it or hate it, shaving is a part of modern daily life. Just make sure you're taking precautions to avoid infection.

YOUR TOOTHBRUSH *and* HOLDER

Bad news. If you have a toothbrush holder, it might well be one of the most germ-infested objects in your entire bathroom! And sorry to say, toothbrushes aren't that far behind.

- A toothbrush picks up the bacteria in your mouth and can stay on the brush if you don't rinse it well enough.

- An average toothbrush can contain millions of bacteria. Fortunately, many of these are already in your mouth and won't hurt you. But traces of things like E. coli and other nasty infectious varieties have been found in many studies.

- If you just lay your toothbrush down on a surface, bacteria still in it will transfer to the surface, vice versa. You're placing a wet object on a surface to dry, which in a bathroom can take ages. In that time, bacteria will take hold and multiply.

- If you use a toothbrush holder or rack, that will help the brush dry out faster, but that water is going to seep down somewhere. And wherever it ends up will become over grown with bacteria in a short time.

Happily, you don't need to abandon brushing your teeth, nor should you!

- Never share your toothbrush with anyone. Ever.

- Always rinse your brush thoroughly after each use. Make sure the water really gets out all the toothpaste and any food particles picked up while brushing.

- Let your toothbrush dry completely between brushings. Don't use a plastic cover over the bristles. This might seem like a good idea, but it can trap moisture, allowing bacteria to flourish.

- Clean your toothbrush once a week in white vinegar. A half cup or so of vinegar makes a great sterilizer. Let your brush sit in it for half an hour. This will kill germs and remove any odors.

- Replace your toothbrush about every three to four months, or more frequently if you've been sick, are immunocompromised, etc. This goes for attachment brushes on electric toothbrushes, as well.

- Use a holder that keeps your brush upright. Water will drip to the bottom of it from the brush, so every couple of days, wipe it down with some disinfectant and keep anything from pooling and building up.

- Keep your holder as far away from the toilet as possible, and remember to always shut the lid of the toilet when you flush. This will prevent any bacteria in aerosol form from landing on your toothbrush. Yes, it can easily happen, and yes, that's gross!

Your toothbrush is essential to good oral and overall health, so make sure it's as clean as can be.

THE TOILET BRUSH

It probably comes as no surprise that the brush you use to scrub your toilet is crawling with germs. And if you put it back into its plastic holder or container after using it, it's going to drip toilet water into the bottom that will be a bacteria party.

- After cleaning, when you lift it out of the toilet, the germs that are on it can drip to the toilet seat (lid up or not), the floor, and anywhere else the water can get to before you replace it. And the tray is going to get contaminated quickly.

- The more you use it, the more the bristles will fray over time, making it less effective in cleaning the toilet. It also means you'll have to scrub harder, which can splash more water and germs around, which means more bacteria get everywhere.

Keeping a toilet brush clean may seem impossible, but there are a few simple things you can do to keep it cleaner, at least.

- Replace the brush every six months or so, or when you can see that the bristles are getting worn. You want this particular cleaning tool to be in great shape when you use it. Think of it like a toothbrush . . . or, don't, actually!

- After cleaning the bowl, it's a good idea to disinfect the brush before putting it back in its holder. This can also extend the life of the brush, though you should still replace it twice a year. With the bowl completely cleaned, give the toilet a flush and let the brush get washed by the flushing water. Just keep your face away from the bowl!

- Now soak the brush in a bucket of a one part bleach to nine- or ten-parts water solution. This will kill any remaining bacteria. Rinse it out again and return to the holder. This will keep dirty toilet water from pooling in the plastic holder.

The toilet brush is essential, but also expendable after a certain amount of time. Be prepared to get a new one twice a year, and keep the one you have as clean as possible.

DOORKNOBS, WINDOWS and ELSEWHERE

This may seem obvious, but the doorknob of your bathroom is going to see a lot of germs. If you've come home and need to use the facilities, and you close the door, you've just touched the handle with your unwashed hands. The next person who comes along and touches the handle, even if their hands are clean, is going to pick up whatever you've left there.

- One study showed that bathroom doorknobs have more microorganisms per square inch than a toilet seat! This isn't surprising, since people are touching them all the time.

- If there are multiple people using the same bathroom (especially children), then each one is contributing their own germs for the next person to pick up. In cold and flu seasons this can be a big problem.

- Did you inadvertently open the window before washing your hands? Then you've just spread germs there, too.

- Did you touch anything else? Guess, what? Germ town!

The solution is simple: just a little regular disinfecting and good hygiene habits will keep these germs at bay.

- Try to keep handles and doorknobs as clean as possible. Wipe them down with a bit of disinfectant every day if you can, especially if there have been several people using the bathroom. Disinfectant wipes or a spray bottle and cloth will work just fine. Make sure to get every part of the handle and let it dry.

- Get in the habit of washing your hands for a good twenty seconds or more with each wash, and make sure that everyone in your family does the same.

- If you've just come home, try not to touch anything in the bathroom until you've washed your hands first. Need to answer nature's call? Wash your hands first, and *then* close the door. Washing before and after using the toilet is a great way to cut down the spread of germs.

Door handles in general can be a problem for harboring bacteria that are only too happy to jump onto the next hand, but in the bathroom, it's even more the case. A regular wiping down of surfaces and good handwashing practices will help stop these germs in their tracks.

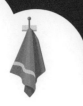

BATH *and* HAND TOWELS

Stepping out of the shower and wrapping yourself in a nice, warm bath towel is one of life's little pleasures. But here's where we ruin it!

- Because they're large, bath towels are usually covered in bacteria. This is even truer if they are damp or hanging in a steamy room, or both. They might never get the chance to dry out fully, and that's just an invitation for all kinds of microorganisms to multiply.

- The good news is that much of these bacteria come from our bodies and are harmless, since we've adapted to them. However . . .

- One study found that almost 90 percent of bathroom towels contained coliform bacteria and nearly 14 percent had E. coli.

- It can be tempting to just leave bath towels up to hang, often for weeks, but if you use and reuse your bath towel often, you're potentially smearing bacteria all over your body when you dry off. And you just got clean!

- If you don't wash your hands properly, any remaining bacteria will just end up hitching a ride on your hand towels.

- Damp towels can be a good home for bacteria, yeast, mold, and even viruses.

- Damp towels are also a potentially dangerous breeding ground for MRSA, which is an infection caused by antibiotic-resistant staphylococcus aureus.

The solution to clean bath towels is simple.

- Wash them in hot water (check the tags for specific instructions). Frequently. Have a dedicated laundry load just for all your towels (kitchen and bathroom) and washcloths. Do this every other day, especially if you have children, or it's cold and flu season, or both. Never let a towel go unwashed for more than a week. Is it stinky? It's well past time for a wash!

- Try to use a detergent with activated oxygen bleach, to really get in and kill those bugs. Just make sure it's color-safe and won't end up stripping colors out of your beloved towels!

- On days when you're not washing, be sure to let towels dry out completely between uses. This greatly reduces the risk of bacteria growing and transmitting. Hang them on a bar, rather than a hook, so that every inch has a chance to dry out fully. Never throw them on the floor, pile them up in a corner, or just drape them over the side of the bath tub.

Regular laundering and making sure to keep your towels dry should do the trick to keep them from becoming germ central in your bathroom, and even worse, rubbing those germs all over yourself after getting clean!

WASHCLOTHS *and* LOOFAHS

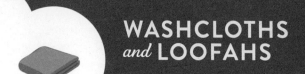

You're not going to want to hear this. Those wonderful loofahs you use? Your favorite shower washcloth? Yeah, they're probably saturated with germs!

- Loofahs may feel good, but they rarely dry out completely, which allows damp dark places for bacteria, yeast, and mold to grow and thrive. They also trap skin cells and dirt, which can be great food for growing bacteria. If you've just shaved your face or legs and rub this germ-encrusted object all over your skin, you run the risk of infection, if anything is hiding in there.

- Most dermatologists now say that using a loofah is not a good idea at all. Sorry, but you might want to let it go.

- Washcloths can also be great incubators for germs, if they are allowed to stay damp.

- If either of these items has bacteria on it and you haven't washed and dried them properly, you're just smearing bacteria all over yourself the next time you take a shower.

Keeping them dry is the key to keeping them germ-free.

- Allow your washcloth to dry out completely between showers. Don't just throw it over the showerhead. It will stay scrunched up and damp, allowing much more bacteria to multiply. Drape it over an empty space on the shower curtain rod, or have a dedicated rack to hang it over.

- Make sure that you use your bathroom fan or open a window, to let out steam and humidity.

- Wash your washcloth in hot water with towels and similar items after every use, or a few days at most. This will keep it much cleaner, fresher, and germ-free.

- Never share a washcloth or a loofah with someone else.

- If you really want to use a loofah, be prepared to replace it with a new one every three to four weeks. Don't just keep using the same one for months or longer!

- If you have an actual luffa plant, it can be disinfected with a one-part bleach to nine-parts water solution. Soak it in this solution for five minutes at least once a week.

When it comes to your shower scrubbers, it's all about avoiding the damp. Make sure that your cloth or loofah has an adequate chance to dry out, and you'll greatly reduce the amount of bacteria.

BAR *and* HAND SOAP

Whether you use soap from a dispenser, or prefer a bar of soap, whether in the shower or at the sink, you're going to come into contact with germs; that's inevitable. But which one is better at keeping germs to a minimum? *Is* one better than the other? The answer is, it depends. If you really prefer one over the other, you probably don't have to switch, but here are a few things to keep in mind.

- Yes, soap bars are covered in germs, but they're mostly your germs, so they're simply things living on your skin that are already there. Washing your hands with your own bar soap doesn't present any real problems.

- Hand soap dispensers will pick up germs from the outside world, especially if you've just come into the bathroom to wash your hands. When you touch the handle, you're potentially transferring whatever you might have picked up outside to it.

It doesn't really matter which kind of soap you use, as long as you take a few simple precautions to help keep the spread of germs to a minimum.

- Clean off your soap dispensers regularly. A disinfectant spray or wipe will do the trick, and help keep outside bacteria from building up.

- When you come in to wash, try not to touch the handle or pump of the soap dispenser with your hands. Use your forearm or even elbow. This will keep your hands from transferring whatever germs are on them to your nice clean soap dispenser.

- Wet your soap bar, and work it into a good lather for fifteen seconds before using it to wash your hands or body. This gives time for the soap's surfactants to lift up germs on the soap's surface and allow them to be washed away.

- In the shower, apply soap directly to your body first, rather than using a washcloth or loofah. Use those to scrub the soap around further after you've applied it.

- Consider not sharing your bar of soap with someone else, especially in the shower. Everyone has their own unique makeup of bacteria, and though it's unlikely, someone else may have some that aren't a problem for them, but could be a problem for you, and vice versa. If you have any cuts or scrapes, it could be an entry point for bacteria into your system. Each member of the household should have their own dedicated soap in a shared shower.

- Try to let bar soaps dry out completely between each use. Get a soap bar holder with slats to allow water to drain off. Don't just let it sit in a dish and trap water underneath it. As we've seen, pooled water is bad for pretty much everything!

- Be sure to clean out the dish regularly, and not let soap scum and residue build up.

Ensuring that your soap stays clean and safe will make sure that its main purpose, to wash away germs, is the only thing you need to worry about.

THE SHOWER MAT

Rubber shower and bathtub mats serve an important function. They help your feet grip the floor of your shower, and drastically reduce the risk of slipping in the soapy water and getting injured. This is no joke. Estimates are that, in the United States, there are several hundred thousand bathroom injuries a year, a good number of them coming from slipping in showers or tubs. This is especially true for older people. So a mat can be essential, but it can also be a major source of bacterial contamination. Cloth mats outside the shower or tub are great for drying off your feet, but they can harbor all kinds of bacteria, too, simply because they're frequently damp.

- Mats tend to have suckers on the bottom, allowing them to grip the tub or shower floor. This is a good thing for preventing falls, but if you don't pull up the mat after every shower or bath, you're leaving a whole miniature world for bacteria to play in, especially on the underside.

- Leaving the mat also allows for soap scum and mineral deposits to build up, leading to a gross, bacteria-infested mess when you do pull it up. Mold is another common feature of bath mat undersides that don't get cleaned often enough.

- If you're using a mat in the bath and haven't cleaned it, all of those bacteria will be only too happy to jump off and have a swim with you.

Keep your mat clean with a few dedicated actions.

- Pull up your bathroom mat after every shower, and have a place to drape it so that it can dry out.

- Once a week, fill your bathtub with hot water and add two cups of bleach. Put your rubber mat in and let it soak in the solution for a good fifteen minutes. If there is visible mold or mildew on the bottom, you can let it soak for up to two hours. Just be sure to open your bathroom window to turn on the ceiling vent or fan to prevent the buildup of bleach fumes.

- Wear rubber gloves and use a scrub brush to scrub away any gunk and mold that might be collecting on it. Clean both sides, and then rinse thoroughly with water.

- For your cloth mat when you step out of the shower, wash with towels in hot water in your washing machine once a week. If your mat is not machine washable, get a new one that is. Check the tag for instructions, and have more than one on hand. It should be completely dry for each new person who uses the shower or bath. Don't put your feet down on a damp mat.

Rubber shower mats can prevent injuries and, sometimes, even save lives. If you need one, cleaning it needs to become a regular part of your daily routine.

SHAMPOO *and* OTHER BOTTLES

Shampoo bottles and other containers that live in the bathroom are subject to damp conditions, usually on a daily basis, which means that their surfaces are great places for bacteria to thrive.

- Water and condensation cover not just your showering bottles (shampoo, conditioner, etc.), but the steam from a hot shower seeps into every corner of the bathroom, leaving behind a wet coating on everything.

- If you leave bottles in the shower or tub after bathing, they can trap little circles of water underneath them, which are basically bacterial public swimming pools.

- Spray bottles filled with water or other liquids can easily become germ factories, especially at the nozzles. And then, every time you use them, you're spraying germs all over yourself.

Keep your bottles cleaner with a few extra precautions.

- Try to dry out your bathroom as soon as possible after a shower or bath. If you have a fan, use it, or open the window. The longer the air stays steamy and damp, the easier it is for bacteria to expand and conquer.

- After the air has cleared, it's a good idea to dry off the bottles you use the most, if condensation is still sticking to them.

- Make sure to wipe down containers for facial creams and such, and always wash your hands before dipping into them. Better yet, have a stash of tongue depressors on hand to scoop out what you need, without having to dip your fingers into the container.

- Don't dilute your shampoo with water to make it last longer. One study tried comparing undiluted and diluted shampoos, with the latter being diluted by 50 percent and 75 percent water each. The amount of bacterial overgrowth in the diluted containers was shocking, while the undiluted shampoo remained pretty much as it had been. Adding the water just added whatever bacteria were already in it to the mix and gave them a perfect place to multiply. While much of these bacteria are harmless, you're essentially dumping them all over your head each time you use diluted shampoo! If your shampoo is a concentrate to be mixed with water (this is often the case with pet shampoos), only mix it when you are ready to use it. Don't mix up a batch and let it sit for days.

- If you have a bottle filled with water (say, for wetting down your hair), don't just let it be in the container for days or weeks; this is a surefire way for bacteria to thrive. Empty it out regularly and wash well in soap and hot water. You can soak the nozzle in a one-part bleach to nine-parts water solution for fifteen minutes once a week, to make sure that nothing is growing there that then gets sprayed on your hair or face.

Keeping your bottles clean is essential to controlling bacterial growth, so don't neglect these little tasks.

THE FLOOR

Let's be honest, the bathroom floor can be quite the mess. All those germs and bacteria floating around in the air or falling off things are going to find a happy home on the floor, and will love attaching themselves to your feet every time you're in there. We deposit dirt and hair, and shed skin every time we're in there, and this adds up pretty quickly. And while the bathroom floor isn't the dirtiest, germiest place in the bathroom (not by a long shot), it can still harbor some unpleasant surprises.

- Studies have shown that staphylococcus and E. coli are common bacteria residing on bathroom floors. If you're wandering in and out of the bathroom with bare feet or socks on, you're picking those up and taking them to the rest of your home. If you wear shoes from outside, you're introducing all kinds of microscopic critters!

- Another study estimated that between 68 and 98 percent of the bacteria on your bathroom floor either comes from your skin (so probably not as much of a problem) or was tracked in from the outside world (could be a bigger problem).

- Even so, fecal bacteria from splashing toilet water can sail through the air and have a happy landing on the floor, where it's only too willing to put down roots.

It should be obvious that keeping the floor clean is an essential part of keeping the whole bathroom clean. But it shouldn't be too much of a chore. Here are some tips.

- Always put the lid of your toilet down before flushing; this prevents an aerosol spray of water droplets and bacteria (the "toilet plume") from flying out and landing on nearby surfaces, including the floor.

- Don't throw dirty clothes or wet towels on the floor and leave them there for hours or days at a time. It's easy for bacteria to grow in damp conditions. Hang up towels to dry and put dirty clothes in a dedicated hamper to be washed and wash them frequently.

- Never wear outside shoes in the bathroom. Put them on before you leave and take them off at the door when you come back.

- Vacuum and then wash the floor, at least once every two weeks, if not more. Vacuuming will pick up dust, hair balls, and skin deposits, while a good mop after will, well, mop up the operation. A standard commercial floor cleaner or a half-water, half-white vinegar mix are both good options for getting the floor spotless and (mostly) germless. Pay special attention to the area around the toilet.

- Clean the floor last, after cleaning everything else. Any dirt, dust, or other grit that you've knocked to the floor (and it will happen!) can then be cleaned up.

Keeping a clean bathroom floor is not a difficult job, and since it is surprisingly lower in germs than many bathroom surfaces, it shouldn't be something that will take too long, if you keep at it on a regular basis.

CHAPTER 4:

GERMS IN THE OUTSIDE WORLD

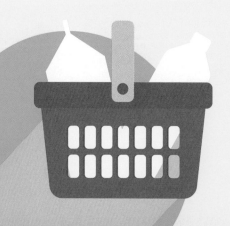

The big, scary, outside world has more germs than you can possibly imagine! They're literally swarming all over everything, and each time you touch a surface of any kind, you'll be picking up countless numbers of unknown bacteria and other hidden life-forms. But remember, the good news is that the vast majority of these are harmless, and some may even be beneficial. But that doesn't mean everything is just fine . . . .

When you are out in the world, you'll also be in contact with untold numbers of people, carrying untold numbers of infectious agents around with them. In order to give yourself the best chance of getting through the world outside your window (which you've cleaned by now, right?) without picking up something you don't want, read this chapter. It has details about the many, many ways you can be exposed to bacteria and viruses all around you, and what you can do about it!

IN YOUR CAR

Your car may not be your castle, but it is a place where you'll likely spend a lot of time, whether you're commuting or just being out and about. This home away from home can be many things from transport to an extra storage facility, but one thing that's certain is that if you and other mammals are spending a decent amount of time in it, it will have germs—a lot of them!

- The average American spends 250 to 300 hours per year in their car, but about one-third of people don't clean their cars more than once a year. Twelve percent said that they *never* clean inside their cars!

- One study found that the average car can have about 700 different strains of bacteria living inside of it at any given time.

- The steering wheel alone has been found to have a large number of colony-forming units: six times more than a typical cell phone screen, and four times more than a public toilet seat.

- If you're eating in your car and drop crumbs or pieces on the floor or they fall into the seat cracks, they become breeding grounds for all kinds of bacteria. Mold, viruses, and pollen can all make their homes in your vehicle, too.

- Germs cover every surface: the gear shift, cupholders, radio dials, seat belts, the dashboard, the rearview mirror, etc. If you're storing reusable shopping bags in the backseat and not washing them after every use, their germs are now your car, too.

Despite all of this unsettling information, you need your car, so what can you do to keep it cleaner and safer?

- Clean your car regularly, at least once a month.

- Get in there and vacuum all the surfaces, just as you would in your home. Vacuuming, combined with dusting and brushing, will remove grit and bigger particles of dirt. Try to get down into the cracks in the seats and don't forget to clean under them.

- If you have cloth seats, consider given them a periodic shampoo. There are products specially made for this, available at most auto stores. Doing this will give your seats a deeper clean and remove stains. For vinyl or leather seats, use an all-purpose cleaner, or one specially formulated for the surface.

- Use spray disinfectant or wipes (or both) on the dashboard and other surfaces. Use a glass cleaner to clean the inside of your windshield and other car windows.

- Don't forget to clean out your trunk, vacuum it, and keep it clean. Don't throw things in there as storage and forget about them.

- Make sure that your air filter is cleaned or replaced as needed to prevent drawing in outside dirt and germs.

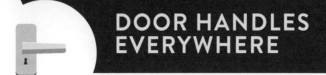

DOOR HANDLES EVERYWHERE

Door handles in your own home are bad enough for spreading germs, but once you get out into the world, it's a whole different ball game, and a much nastier one!

Any place and every place has doors, and most of them have handles, latches, or knobs. And that means that anyone and everyone are touching them throughout the day. They may be cleaned at night (or not), but that doesn't prevent an appalling number of germs building up every day through regular use.

- Some handles, such as outside ones that people use to enter a building, will be much germier than others. Hospital handles might well be among the worst.

- One study, using a dummy version of norovirus in an office, found that by applying it to door handles, it spread to between 40 and 60 percent of the people there in only two hours. So, if you want to know how colds and the flu travel around so fast, there's a great example!

- Most viruses die within twenty-four to forty-eight hours of arriving on a surface like a door handle, but some bacteria, such as MRSA, can last for weeks. Another strain, *C. difficile*, was found to survive for up to five months.

- In general, public door handles can harbor two to three times the amount of germs as surfaces such as shopping carts, faucets, and even cell phones.

Well, that's not good news! So, what can you do to stay safe, or at least safer?

- Wash your hands frequently with soap and warm water. This is still the best advice, especially during cold and flu season.

- When washing your hands in a public restroom, be mindful that if you've just cleaned your hands, but then turn off the faucet (unless it automatically shuts off) or touch the door handle, you'll be picking up a new batch of germs on your newly clean hands. If there are paper towels, grab one and use it to turn off the faucet. Use another to open the door; throw it in the bin as you leave the bathroom. The point is to keep from recontaminating your hands.

- In your office, you might want to keep a box of disinfectant wipes and use them on the door handles that you are touching regularly.

- When you're out in the world and you need to open doors (which may be often), be careful about touching your face, especially your eyes and mouth, after opening any door. Always try to wash your hands again as soon as possible.

Adding a few new practices to your daily routine should be enough to minimize the risk that is every door handle in sight!

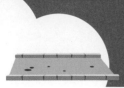

THE SIDEWALK

The average city or town sidewalk is awash in germs from just about everything you can imagine: shoes, fallen food, garbage, feces, urine, vomit, animals tracking all kinds of substances across the pavement, and so on. Everything and everyone wanders across these well-worn paths at one time or another, and they're not cleaned nearly as often as they should be. Even a good rainstorm will not always wash everything away.

If you can imagine it, it's on a sidewalk, somewhere. Probably in your town. Ew. All the bacteria, all the viruses, all the everything are going to be lying in wait out there, ready for you to step on (or in) them and bring them home. Just think about how many people walk on a busy sidewalk in any given day, and you'll understand just how easily germs are shed and picked up.

You can't avoid sidewalks. Fortunately, there are some simple things you can do to keep all those little life-forms from hitching a ride home with you.

- Again, forget the "five second rule." If you drop a bit of food on the sidewalk, it's gone. That's it. Say your good-byes. Any number of germs will attach themselves to it instantly, and you don't want those anywhere near you!

- If you drop clothing or another item on the sidewalk, try to keep it separate and wash it as soon as possible when you get home. While it's unlikely that you'll pick up anything really bad, but taking precautions is always a good idea.

- Remove your shoes as soon as you get home and have a dedicated place to keep them. Never walk around inside your home with all of the day's germs on your shoe soles; you'll be tracking them and depositing them everywhere! Look into options for washing your shoes and keeping them clean.

- Obviously, if you've stepped in anything at all (gum, food, or even worse), leave your shoes outside until you can clean them.

- If possible, don't bring your bicycle into your home. Its rubber tires will track germs into your home as easily as your shoes. If it can be safely stored outside, great. If not, spray the tires with some disinfectant and let sit for a few minutes before bringing the bike inside. Try to store it in a place that won't be in the way (and definitely not in the kitchen!); keep the floor around it extra clean. If you can mount your bike on a wall hook or rack, even better!

Whether you're out running, jogging, walking, or biking, you're going to pick up all kinds of things from your local sidewalks. Just be sure not to bring them inside!

GROCERY STORES

In the age of COVID-19, going to the grocery store has become quite the chore for many. It's frustrating, but most of us have learned to live with it as a small sacrifice to help stop the spread of a dangerous disease. But even without these contemporary concerns, stores of all kinds, and grocery stores in particular, are veritable germ havens.

- The fruit and veggies in the produce aisle can be bathing in germs. One study found that the average item had up to 700 times the number of bacteria as a car steering wheel.

- The meat and fish aisle? The products there are positively swimming in germs and bacteria than can easily transfer to your hands and to other items in your cart.

- Remember how bad tablets and cell phones are for harboring germs? Well, fridge doors in the frozen aisle have been shown to have over 1,200 times more bacteria than the surface of a cell phone!

- Among the more common types of grocery store germs are gram-positive cocci, which are associated with all sorts of conditions, from strep throat to staph infections, and even blood poisoning.

- Upscale markets and stores have been found to have up to thirty times more positive bacteria colonies than some regular stores, possibly due to organic food and the lack of pesticides. Good for you in one way, not so good in another!

- Budget grocery stores were the worst of all. Some surfaces tested revealed 5.5 million bacteria colonies per square inch!

- Self-checkout and credit card touch screens harbor just about anything. One study showed that 50 percent of touch screens had traces of antibiotic-resistant MRSA, more than would be found in most hospitals.

Wow, that's a lot of germs! Here are some ways to minimize what you transmit and pick up while shopping for food.

- Always buy produce that is not cracked or split open anywhere. Yes, you will have to touch and examine them before choosing, but at least you'll be buying items that don't have openings that could allow for bacteria and germs to enter.

- Always wash all produce thoroughly before use at home. Wash your own hands first, for at least twenty seconds. Rinse produce before peeling, and gently rub with your clean hands or a gentle scrub brush. You can use special soaps or vegetable cleaners, but they're not necessary. Dry with a paper towel.

- You should always double-bag meat and fish sold in packages, to prevent any juices from leaking out onto your other groceries.

- Be sure to use hand sanitizer after shopping and give your hands a good wash as soon as you get home.

- Wash reusable bags after each use; otherwise, bacteria can sit in the bottom and grow, and hop onto your next batch of groceries.

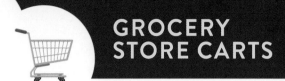

GROCERY STORE CARTS

One particular concern for many since 2020 is the safety of shopping carts. People have become much more aware of the need for clean handles, and the fact that these are touched over and over by multiple people throughout the day. The thing is, even before COVID-19, this was a problem that more people should have been taking seriously.

- One study showed that a sampling of eighty-five grocery store carts had a far greater amount of bacteria than public restrooms.

- Among the bacteria found were campylobacter and salmonella. More than half also contained E. coli.

- There were up to 138,000 total bacteria per square inch of cart handle.

- Studies have also shown that bacteria increase throughout the day, as more people use and reuse carts.

- Wipe-downs and sanitizing efforts definitely reduced the amount of bacteria, but didn't eliminate all of it.

Fortunately, most stores have taken appropriate actions to reduce the risk of transmission of viruses and other infectious agents.

- As of 2020–21, most stores are sanitizing their carts after each use. This is a good thing, as simple alcohol-based sanitizers (of 70 percent alcohol or more) are good at killing viruses and bacteria on contact. If your local stores are doing this (and they probably are), this is good.

- You may want to opt in for some extra protection. Many stores also offer hand sanitizer for their customers, in spray or gel forms. Use this before and after handling a store cart. Get a squirt on the way in, and one on the way out! Also, keep some sanitizer in your car and use it after shopping.

- You can also opt to wear latex or other gloves for an extra layer of protection. This is probably not necessary for everyone, but those with compromised immune systems or other health problems may wish to protect themselves further.

- Go to the store earlier in the day, rather than later, if you can. Fewer people will have touched the carts, even if they are cleaned throughout the day.

- Always wash your hands thoroughly as soon as you can after handling a shopping basket or cart.

Overall, shopping carts have become much safer since 2020. This is a good thing in general, and it's a practice that should continue well into the future.

FREE FOOD SAMPLES

Because of COVID-19, almost all grocery and specialty stores have stopped offering free food samples, which used to be a staple. This section is written on the assumption that at some point, it will be safe to resume food sampling, coffee and wine tasting, etc.

- Like buffets (see later in this chapter), you have no idea how long foods set out for sampling have been sitting there. If the store has just opened, or is busy, it will be fresh, since there will be a rapid turnover. But a relatively empty store where the samples are just sitting there? Who knows? And meat and dairy that are not properly stored may already have bacteria that are beginning to multiply.

- Who else has touched the food? In theory, no one, and those who put it out often wear protective gloves (as they should), but you can't guarantee that someone with dirty, unwashed hands didn't pick up something and then set it back down again when no one was looking. Is this paranoid? Perhaps, but you can do an online search for food sample horror stories and find all sorts of unpleasant examples! Honestly, you probably don't want to do this.

- Various store chains have had recent issues with E. coli outbreaks and other infections in their food samples.

So, should you give up trying out free food samples for good?

- Yes. Yes, you probably should. Tempting as they are, there is probably too much risk, even without pandemic concerns. You simply have no way of knowing who has touched what before you.

- This advice also goes for grocery store buffets, by the way. They can be convenient, but they're probably not very safe, and you should consider other ideas for lunch.

- If you're determined to try samples anyway, make sure the food is set out as you're watching. It will be fresher and you can be sure that no one else has touched it. Get there early or when it is busy so that the food is fresh and quickly turned around. The more people waiting for samples, the more likely the food will be fresh, since they will be turning it out regularly to meet demand.

- Examine how the food is stored. Is hot food kept in a pot to keep it warm? Is cold food refrigerated or kept on ice? If food that's supposed to be cold is just sitting out (unless you see it being placed there), give it a miss.

- How is it served? Do the servers wear gloves? If not, consider not eating it.

- Try to sample only those foods that are served with a plastic fork or spoon. Don't take anything that you have to try by hand; who knows how many others have reached for it with their grubby fingers!

- Give meat and dairy samples a miss. Stick with things like crackers and cookies.

OTHER STORES

Grocery stores aren't the only place where germs are lying in wait to get at you. Oh, no, there are many other locations where germs are lying in wait to attack, hitch a ride, and be a general nuisance.

- Shopping malls and places where large numbers of people gather can be a huge problem, especially during cold and flu season.

- Door and escalator handles, elevator buttons, etc., are all places that viruses and bacteria love to hide out. One touch of any of them, and you've picked up whatever someone else left behind.

- A shopping mall floor is teeming with germs, tracked in from outside by everyone that's walked on it (remember those sidewalks?). These floors are probably only cleaned at night, and usually then, it's just a quick mopping.

- Food courts at shopping malls are risky, especially at busy times. See the section on buffets below for a list of similar risks.

- Tests on public ATMs showed that *each key* can contain thousands of germs.

- Fitting rooms are generally safe, but the clothes you try on may not be. If they'd been tried on by others and put back (a distinct possibility), anything lingering there (yeast infections, bacteria, fecal matter) can transfer to you. New clothes aren't all that new, it turns out!

- Gadget stores, computer shops, and electronics stores have hundreds of people trying out the devices, and all of them are leaving behind germs that can transfer to others.

So, how to best protect yourself?

- As always, keep your hands clean. Wash them often (as often as you can) while you're out, and bring hand sanitizer with you. If you're opening a lot of store doors, you need to be especially mindful of this. And keep your hands away from your face.

- Keep in mind the basic advice about using public restrooms safely (see the next section).

- When trying on clothing, always wear full underwear, and make sure any cuts or abrasions are fully bandaged and covered. If you buy new clothing, wash it as soon as you can. Never wear it before washing. Wash your hands after trying on any items of clothing.

- Keep hand sanitizer with you, especially if you are going into a computer, phone, or device store and are going to try out items.

- Touch screens and credit card machines are swarming with germs, since they're touched so often. You may not be able to wipe one down while you're using it, but try to clean your hands afterward if you can. Do this every time you use any demonstration device.

Shopping can be stressful or fun, depending on your approach. Don't let the multitude of germs add to your worries or ruin the experience!

PUBLIC TOILETS

What can be said about public toilets? Too much, and a lot that you probably don't want to know. Public toilets are not only as germy as your fear they are, they're probably much worse! The good news is that many of these germs are harmless, but it still pays to be cautious.

- Among the things found in public toilets after tests are streptococcus, shigella bacteria, staphylococcus, E. coli, Hepatitis A virus, cold and flu viruses, and sexually transmitted organisms. Yikes!

- Toilet faucets and handles can be covered in germs, since everyone is turning on the tap after doing their business and leaving those germs there for the next person. And if you turn the tap off after washing your hands, you're just picking up all those things again.

- Interestingly, toilet seats are not a good place for passing along germs. Things like STDs don't live for long on seats and have no way to enter your body; your skin is a natural barrier. Some studies even suggest that toilet seat protectors make things worse, but the jury is still out on that one.

- Toilet seat protectors and toilet paper that are not properly protected from the toilet plume spray of each flush will more likely be contaminated.

- Most public toilets don't have lids, so when you flush, a spray of water and bacteria is launched into the air in tiny particles, which are only too happy to stick to your clothing, your face, and wherever else they can alight. Lovely.

- Stall handles have been touched by everyone who's just finished but not yet washed their hands. Door handles are the same, since a lot of people, apparently, don't bother to wash their hands before leaving. Yuck.

So, is this massive petri dish a place you should avoid at all costs? Well, there are some things you can do to make your time in a public restroom safer.

- Always wash your hands thoroughly before leaving. Your tap may have handles, or the faucet may turn off automatically (those are preferred, since they also save water). If you have to turn off the taps by hand, grab a paper towel and keep your hand covered while you do so.

- The same thing goes for door handles when leaving. Use another paper towel to grab the handle; throw it away as you leave.

- When flushing, try to leave the stall just as you flush to avoid a bacterial spray. Flush with your foot, if you can. Some toilets have automatic flushing, because some people don't seem to bother to flush (seriously, who *are* these people?). This is good for keeping the toilet clean but subjects you to a water and bacteria spray that you can't avoid.

- If you have some disinfectant wipes with you, you can always wipe down the seat before sitting down.

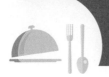

RESTAURANTS

Many restaurants are offering takeout only services, or seating outside, in an attempt to slow the spread of COVID-19. This section is created with the assumption that at some point, restaurants will be opening again as normal.

We all love going out to eat from time to time, whether simple fast food, or something more lavish and elaborate. But being in restaurants is also a great way to come into contact with all kinds of infectious agents.

- Restaurant door handles have been touched by untold numbers of people.

- All restaurants have bathrooms. Many people who use them don't wash their hands properly, or at all.

- Menus are just bad. Think about it: everyone before you and everyone after you will handle a menu. Menus are usually made of paper or cardboard (some are plastic coated). So, all the germs, viruses, bacteria, you name it, are sitting there waiting to hop onto another set of hands at the next available opportunity.

- While dishes and utensils are (we hope!) cleaned in a dishwasher, condiment bottles (salt, pepper, ketchup, soy sauce, etc.), are cleaned less often. When empty, they should be put in a dishwasher, but maybe they'll just be refilled. You have no way of knowing.

- Tables are usually just wiped down between patrons, and often not thoroughly cleaned.

- In some restaurants, chairs are also rarely, if ever, cleaned.

- Those lemon slices some restaurants put in your water? One study found that more than 70 percent of them had harmful microorganisms, which means that they're floating away into your drinking water for a good swim.

- Restaurant floors can get covered with food bits and germs quickly.

Still want to enjoy dining out? Here's how to be safer.

- Always wash your hands before and after eating. Wash your hands again or use hand sanitizer after handling a menu.

- Consider having some disposable disinfectant wipes to give the condiment bottles a rub before using. You'll be doing yourself and the next customer a favor! Or wrap a napkin around condiments bottles and jars and hold them with this barrier.

- Ask for water without lemon, or ask for a slice on the side, so that you can squeeze the juice in yourself, and not just dunk the whole thing in your drink.

- Bearing in mind the state of a typical restaurant floor, remove your shoes as soon as you get home, and don't track germs inside.

BUFFETS

This probably won't surprise you, but there's some bad news about buffets: they're an amazingly good way to spread germs of all kinds! Here are some points to consider.

- The food can sit out for a long time, often for hours. This means it can start to host bacteria, even if it's heated. If you're coming to a buffet at 4:00 p.m. that's been going since noon, you're taking a bigger risk. Salad bars are even more of a problem, since they are just sitting out, even if they have some ice or other means of cooling them.

- Other people have touched the food. This is inevitable. Even if you're being careful, others will likely have touched bread and similar items with their hands. And while buffets often have some kind of shielding over the food, someone will have coughed or sneezed. They just will.

- Cross-contamination happens, even with food that is stored separately in different trays and slots. Some people will use the same utensil for different foods, even though they're not supposed to. This can spread germs, but also causes problems for food allergies. For people with serious allergies, this is no joke.

- The tongs and spoons have been touched by numerous people. Have they all washed their hands properly before touching these? Are you sure? Of course you're not, which means that any bacteria from their hands will to transfer to those utensils for the next person to pick up.

- Trays can be incredibly contaminated. If a buffet has cafeteria-like trays, these need to be thoroughly washed and sterilized after each use. But there's no guarantee that they are.

- A recent Japanese study tried painting a man's hand with an invisible, nontoxic, paint, and then had him dine with nine other people at a buffet for thirty minutes. A black light held up to each after showed that all nine had picked up traces of the paint, and three of them had it on their faces. The paint was also all over clothing, serving utensils, and elsewhere. Imagine if that were a cold or flu virus, or some dangerous bacteria, and you can see how quickly and widely these things can spread!

If you're still determined to take advantage of that all-you-can-eat special, here are a few tips.

- Consider going when the buffet has just opened and food is still being put out. If you can grab food items just as they come out of the kitchen, you'll avoid germs from other people and bacteria that might grow on the food over time. Also, far fewer people will have touched the tongs and spoons.

- Alternately, try to go when the buffet is busy. This may seem counterproductive, but it means that the food will be used up and turned over more quickly. In an empty buffet, the food may sit for far longer. Just be sure to have some hand sanitizer with you before you start eating. Also, wash your hands both before and after eating.

BARS *and* PUBS

Bars and pubs have a limited opening capacity during a pandemic, but even without those concerns, they can still be places where germs love to run amok.

- Spilled drinks on tables and floors create damp and sticky environments, even when they're cleaned up (especially so, if a wet mop runs over the area), which allow perfect places for bacteria to take hold.

- Tables and the main bar are sometimes just wiped down with damp towels, which actually can spread bacteria around even more.

- Glasses should be clean, but it's not uncommon for them to be less than ideal, simply because the dishwasher has to clean a lot of them quickly.

- Bar snacks, like nuts. In open bowels where people can dip their fingers into them. Enough said.

- Bars are often crowded, filled with people breathing all over each other, even if unintentionally. Germs and viruses float about freely in the air, to be inhaled by anyone who comes by.

- The usual concerns about germ-coated restrooms, menus, and tables are just as common in bars as restaurants.

So, are your bar days over? There are some things you can do to make drinking out a safer experience.

- Avoid the free snacks. Sorry, but you just don't know where they've been. Even if you get a clean, fresh bowl, the snacks themselves may have been sitting in a contaminated container for who knows how long.

- Avoid the fruit garnishes: lemons, limes, cherries, unless you can see that they are stored safely. They can add flavor and color, but they could also be harboring untold amounts of bacteria and anything else. If they've not been refrigerated, or are sitting in containers on the bar, it's even worse. Further, you have no idea of knowing if they've been washed, or if the cutting board they were chopped on has been washed.

- Try to avoid drinks with ice. In a lot of bars, the ice buckets are kept at hip level, which means any number of things can dip into them or be spilled. Further, ice machines have been found to be filled with bacteria like E. coli and other lovely things. One study suggested that the ice machine they looked at was dirtier than toilet water!

- Keep an eye out for dirty glasses and other signs that things aren't being cleaned properly.

- Watch out for how glasses are handled by staff. Are they picking them up by the rim? That's not sanitary. Also, observe where the glasses are stored. They should really have their own dedicated storage rack or space.

NIGHTCLUBS

A nightclub may be the last place you're interested in going, or it may be the first. Nightclubs are on hold in most places right now due to COVID-19, but at some point, if you're itching to get back out on the dance floor, do so, but go back in armed with new knowledge about the other risks that being in an enclosed space with many people can bring. And yes, it's risky!

- Lots of people in close quarters in a hot environment are breathing heavily and filling the air with loads of germ-laden aerosols in their breath, constantly. This, combined with the poor ventilation and lack of windows can mean that the air easily carries viruses, such as the common cold, the flu, etc. You're breathing it all in.

- Viruses aren't the only concern. One nightclub in Germany recently reported an outbreak of bacterial meningitis. Other types of dangerous bacteria have been found in all the usual places: restrooms, tabletops, chairs, bars and bar glasses, etc.

- Your protection from bacteria and other infectious agents is entirely down to the hygiene habits of the several hundred people around you. It's a sure bet that not all of them are washing their hands properly, and all it takes are a few coughs or sneezes for germs to get out on the dance floor and party with everyone else!

So, are your clubbing days over? They might be, sorry to say.

- Nightclubs, like gyms, are prime grounds for harboring, breeding, and spreading germs. While these places are usually frequented by the young and the healthy, that's no guarantee of immunity from whatever might be there. Take stock of your own health and ask if it's worth the risk.

- As always, bring some disinfectant wipes and use them to quickly wipe down surfaces before touching them, especially in restrooms, or at tables where you might be sitting.

- If you have the option, use some form of contactless payment for drinks, rather than handing over and accepting cash (see later in this chapter). This is far more sanitary and won't require you to handle cash that's been touched by everyone who uses it before you.

- Wash your hands. Frequently. And be careful who you bump up against.

This may seem like a downer section, but nightclubs are best left to the young and vibrant, those whose immune systems are strong, and can put up with the full-on germ assault that these venues can bring.

HOTELS *and* MOTELS

There's something satisfying about checking into a nice hotel room: everything is cleaned, the sheets are fresh, the bed is made, you're in a new location, and you can't wait to get a good night's sleep. The only problem is, there are a whole lot of microorganisms sharing the room with you that will be only too happy to jump on you and show their appreciation for their new visitor. Here are the uncomfortable facts.

- Hotel rooms aren't nearly as clean as they might seem, even when they've been vacuumed and straightened up.

- Turnover in hotel rooms can be rapid, often mere hours between guests, so a thorough cleaning is often not possible if the staff is in a rush.

- Some things likely not to be cleaned between check-ins include TV remote controls, drapes, chairs, unused mugs, refrigerator door handles, room door handles, and even the bathtub, beyond a quick rinse.

- While sheets are usually changed daily (usually!), bedspreads, blankets, and covers can go for weeks, even months without being cleaned. Sorry to say, that snuggly cover may have the germs of dozens, or even hundreds, of guests on it! This also goes for extra blankets in the closet, and extra pillows. Even if they've been used, they might just get folded up and put back in the closet again.

- If the previous guest had a head cold and sneezed in the room, the virus can linger on surfaces for up to forty-eight hours, or longer.

166

- Are your bathroom sink handles disinfected? Are you sure?

- Desks and countertops are often just given a quick wipe-down (if the staff are in a hurry to get the room turned over), and even then, the same towel that cleaned the bathroom might be used.

It should be obvious now that it's inevitable you're going to come into contact with hotel germs. So what can you do to minimize the risk?

- Bring disinfectant wipes with you and run a couple over the sink and shower taps, toilet handle, door handle, coffee maker, TV remote, etc., just as a precaution. Basically, if you're going to touch it, disinfect it first.

- Some experts suggest never using the bedspread at all. Take it off and chuck it over a chair or fold it back to the edge of the bed. Some hotels now use covers that are more washable. If you're in doubt, ask the front desk.

- Avoid using glassware and even coffee mugs. Sorry to say, in some hotels, these are simply rinsed out and put back on the table, rather than being run through a dishwasher. Yeah, that's gross, but it does happen.

- Wash your hands frequently, especially after entering and before leaving a room.

Hotels are an essential part of travel, and whether for business or pleasure, you will have to use them at some time or another. Just make sure to use them safely!

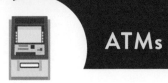

ATMs

While more and more people are going paperless, ATMs are still useful when you need a bit of extra cash or want to deposit a check. There's just one problem: germs, of course! As you can probably imagine, a machine being touched by loads of people every day is not going to be the cleanest thing in the world.

- A recent study of twenty different ATMs across New York City found that in general, they were dirtier than the handle on a toilet in a public restroom, or a pole on a New York subway car.

- However, the same study showed that surfaces like restaurant door handles and escalator handles had significantly more germs and bacteria, probably because they are handled by more people even more often.

- Indoor ATMs, such as those in stores, tend to have more bacteria on them than outdoor ones. This is especially true in grocery stores and other food outlets.

- The worst part of the ATM is usually the card reader, not the keypad. This may have to do with so many germ-infested cards sliding in and out of the machine, and bacteria hopping on and off like it's a microscopic bus terminal! So, even if your card is disinfected and clean before you put it in, it will almost certainly be coated in a new layer of bacteria when the machine spits it back out.

- ATMs near food stores, cafes, and restaurants can also harbor mold and foodborne illnesses.

How do you use ATMs safely?

- Again, always wash your hands as soon as possible after using a public ATM.

- Consider wearing a disposable or washable glove or using a tissue over your fingers when typing in your PIN or touching the screen.

- Bear in mind that your card will come back out of the reader with a new host of germs, so if you just throw it back in your wallet, they might well take up residence there. Consider having small plastic bag or some such to put in into instead, and wash it or disinfect it when you get home. Or, keep a pack of disinfectant wipes with you and clean your card before putting it back into your wallet or card case.

The ATM is still a useful device for many. Just be sure you're using it safely!

STORE CREDIT CARD MACHINES

More and more, people are going paperless, and ditching cash in favor of the convenience of cards, or even using their phones. Considering how many germs can live on a typical dollar bill of any denomination, this seems wise. Less contact with something that's been handled by countless people before you is a good idea, right? Yes, it is, but here comes the bad news: credit cards and the machines that process them aren't much better!

- Every time you put a credit card on a restaurant table or in a tray, it's being exposed to whatever was there before it.

- If you have to give your card to someone, they're touching it along with every other card they've had that day, allowing for an easy transfer of germs.

- A recent study of the number of germs on cards found that they actually have *more* germs of all kinds than coins and paper money!

- Staphylococcus and salmonella were the bacteria types frequently found on cards, especially those used in eateries. Staphylococcus was also found in wallets, presumably having hitched a ride there from the cards.

- When you punch in your PIN or other information, whether at a keypad or on a touch screen, you're touching what untold numbers of people have touched before. These screens and areas are often not cleaned frequently (though in the age of COVID-19, that may no longer be true in many establishments).

So, if you want to go (or stay) cashless, what can you do?

- Wash your hands before and after using your card and a card machine.

- Chip cards tend to have a somewhat lower number of germs than swipe cards.

- Clean your card(s) regularly. You can use a disinfectant wipe or spray a small amount on a cotton ball and give both sides a good wipe. The magnetic strip is water-resistant and usually safe to gently clean, but you probably don't want to submerge it in water.

- Many card companies now offer the contactless tap-and-go option, which brings your card into far less contact with germ-harboring surfaces. You may want to consider this, if it's available for you.

- Phones that have digital wallet options, like those from Apple Pay, Samsung Pay, or Google Pay, are another way to pay without touching much of anything.

- Online checkout may also be an option for some purchases. If you're ordering food for delivery, you can pay online and never have to use your card at all.

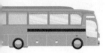

BUSES

Buses and coaches are still a vital part of the American transport system, even though everyone is expected to have a car and use it as much as possible. In big cities, driving your own car may not be as feasible as taking a bus. In a more rural area, the bus may be a vital service for many. But here are some sobering thoughts.

- The benches at bus stops are, in most cases, never cleaned. Ever.

- Everything on a bus, the door, the handrails, and the seats (especially if they are cloth), are covered in germs. Many of these microbes are harmless, but there's no way to know which is which when you sit down.

- Buses are usually cleaned at night, but this might be nothing more than vacuuming and sweeping. Many bus companies do deeper interior cleans, but usually only once every few weeks. Some may go as long as six weeks between these deep cleans, giving plenty of time for bacteria to accumulate and grow, and viruses to live for a few days.

Clearly, buses are not the cleanest of environments, unless you happen to board one the morning after a good deep clean. Here are some tips to make your bus trip safer and more hygienic.

- Given the lack of cleaning that goes on at most bus stops, you may want to stand up while waiting for your bus. Unless you have a genuine need to sit down, try to avoid bus stop benches.

- Check the seat before sitting down. Is it soiled, or does it have anything on it that looks suspect? Try to find another seat, if you can. If it's crowded and there are no other seats, consider standing, if possible.

- Likewise, if a fellow traveler looks sick, and is coughing or sneezing, try to find another seat. It's not being rude; it's just being cautious! If there are no other seats, choose to stand instead, if you can.

- Keep a small bottle of hand sanitizer with you and use it after you sit down. You may want to use a bit more after you get off at your destination.

- Keep your bag or backpack in your lap, if you can. Don't set it on the floor, or even the seat next to you, if possible.

- The advice for riding on trains and subways (see the next section) is equally useful for riding on buses and longer-trip coaches.

The bus is a vital form of transport for short and long journeys. If you're boarding one daily, or even occasionally, just make sure that you take appropriate precautions.

TRAINS *and* SUBWAYS

Trains and subways are essential in many cities for commuters and people needing to get around. While then United States doesn't have the extensive reliance on train systems that Europe has, trains and subway systems won't be going away anytime soon. And neither will their germs!

- One study showed that if you hold a handrail on the New York subway, you can pick up as much bacteria as if you'd shaken hands with *10,000* people! The sheer number of people using these transport systems is astounding, and pretty much every surface will have a multitude of bacteria and other germs on them. Card systems, ATMs, tokens, turnstiles: they're all coated in the bacteria of the thousands that touch them daily.

- Bacteria that have been found on subway surfaces include gram-positive and gram-negative strains, yeasts of all kinds (especially those associated with food), and bacillus.

- Fortunately, most of these microbes are harmless, and less dangerous than even those in our own gut (a lot of them are already there). But that doesn't mean they all are. One study in San Francisco found fecal and flesh-eating bacteria!

- Of the major transport systems in the United States, New York's was by far the germiest, followed by the San Francisco Bay Area's BART system, and then the systems in Chicago and Boston (which was judged the cleanest of those studied).

How do you keep (mostly) germ-free when riding in a car that's visited by so many people on a daily basis?

- Keep a supply of hand sanitizer with you, and try to use it after touching anything like handrails or loops, using the ticket machine, etc. You may want to sanitize more than once on your trip.

- Try to sit in less crowded cars at one end or the other. If it's commute time and this isn't possible, try to find the emptiest car you can. Many people like to crowd into the middle cars, which brings you into contact with many more people touching surfaces and breathing the same air. If you are able to stand in a moving car, consider that option. Then you only need to sanitize your hands from gripping the pole or handle.

- If you have a bag that you need to set down on the train car floor, be sure to clean it with some disinfectant when you get home. Don't just drop it on your home's floor, or worse, the couch. Train floors are covered in germs from shoes.

- Consider not using your phone. Yes, this may be difficult if you have a long trip, but if you're touching handles and then your phone screen, those germs are going to transfer right over to it. At least rub your hands with sanitizer first, and wipe down your screen.

Trains of all kinds are still a vital part of American daily transportation. If you use them, be sure to use them safely.

TAXIS, RENTALS, *and* RIDE-SHARES

These days, ride-share services are everywhere, and whether they are loved or loathed, there's no denying that they're used all the time. They've edged out taxis as the main form of paid private transport, though taxis aren't quite dead yet. The problem, of course, is that with the vast numbers of people getting in and out of them, there's no telling who was in there before you and what they might have left behind, and we're not talking about their wallets!

- Ride-share cars, such as those from Uber and Lyft, are actually far dirtier than taxis or rental cars. One study showed that ride-share vehicles had over six million colony-forming units per square inch. Rental cars had just over two million, while taxis had just over 27,000. None of these are good numbers, but clearly, ride-shares are the worst.

- The germiest areas in ride-shares were seat belts, door handles, and window buttons, while in rentals, germs have been found to be more concentrated on gear shifts, and steering wheels. Taxis had the highest proportion of germs on their seat belts.

- Drivers for ride-shares may or may not clean their vehicle regularly, and you don't really have any way of knowing unless you ask. And that's probably going to sound a bit weird.

- The average ride-share car can transport twenty to thirty passengers a day; that's a lot of germs that accumulate!

Is ride sharing just too dangerous to keep doing?

- It might be, yes. Consider taking a taxi instead. Many of them are required to maintain vehicles to a certain standard, which can include regular cleanings. This may or may not explain why they seem to be less germy than private ride-share vehicles. Still, Uber and Lyft maintain that keeping vehicles clean is a part of their overall policy, and drivers can be penalized or lose their status if they don't keep their cars clean.

- If you do hire a ride-share car, use hand sanitizer after leaving the vehicle. You will have touched the handles and the seat belt at least, so make sure to clean your hands as soon as you can afterward.

- The issue of germs is being discussed by companies and auto manufacturers, and there is a chance that cleaner vehicles will be coming, either by design or with more cleanable surfaces.

- For rentals, it doesn't hurt to wipe down the steering wheel and gear shift with some disinfectant when you first get in, even though it might have been cleaned pretty well before you rent it.

Rentals are still essential when traveling, and there are times when a taxi or ride-share is the only thing you can use to get where you need to go. Use them as you need but be aware that they're probably not as clean as they look and react accordingly.

AIRPORTS

Airports are the beginning or the end of a journey, and thousands of people congregate in them every day to go somewhere, come from somewhere else, and pass through. With that load of people, especially at international airports, every kind of germ imaginable has the possibility of finding its way into the terminals. If you're traveling, you'll potentially be subjected to an untold number of things you'd rather not be subjected to.

- One study showed that the trays in the security line had more bacteria of all kinds than anywhere else in the terminal. And it's the one area you can't avoid in an airport.

- Rhinovirus (the cause of the common cold) was the most frequently found virus in the airport environment, especially at security checkpoints and passport control. This is to be expected, but it doesn't make it any better if you and up catching a cold!

- One study found E. coli, klebsiella, and acinetobacter inside the plastic bins in the TSA security line. These are all fecal bacteria.

- Door handles, public toilets, escalator handles, trays, waiting area seats, etc., will all potentially have bacteria and viruses all over them.

- Food courts can harbor all sort of germs, from the trays for food to the credit card readers.

How do you stay healthy in a place that's so well suited for the spread of germs, and that's visited by thousands of people every day?

- Wash your hands frequently, especially after you get through security. You have literally no idea who's been there before you, or what they might have been unknowingly carrying. Head for the nearest restroom and give them a good wash. Just be sure to observe good restroom hygiene as well!

- Approach every surface with some caution. You can't wipe down everything before you touch it but try to minimize your contact with things.

- If possible, wash your hands after touching food trays and credit card machines and before eating. If you're traveling with others, for example, someone else can watch food while you go wash, and you can take turns. If you're on your own, break out the hand sanitizer after setting your tray down, but before digging into your food.

- Avoid touching your face (especially your eyes or mouth) until you've had a chance to wash your hands.

- Keep up to date with your flu shot; it's a small thing but it can greatly minimize your risk when traveling. There's a good chance that somewhere along the journey someone will have some kind of flu and can potentially pass it on.

There's no way to avoid contact with germs of all kinds in an airport. But a few extra measures can reduce your risk of contracting anything bad and ruining your trip.

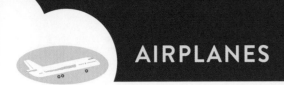

AIRPLANES

Many people love the lure of travel, of getting on a plane and going to faraway places. Unfortunately, when you get on a plane, you're boarding a massive vehicle that has transported hundreds, even thousands, of people before you, and though the insides are cleaned in between flights, there's no way these cleanings can do a thorough job. And that means countless numbers of germs are hitching a ride alongside you.

- Test of interiors have shown some disturbing findings: staphylococcus, E.coli, and MRSA were all present, and in dangerous amounts.

- The MRSA bacteria were present for 168 hours (about a week) on a cloth seatback pocket. E. coli stayed around for 96 hours (about four days) on an airplane armrest.

- So, no matter how well the plane was cleaned, these bacteria were simply not being removed. And even when they died off, they could easily be replaced by new passengers boarding the plane a day or two later.

- Seats, tray tables, armrests, window shades, in-flight magazines, and toilet handles are all places where unwanted bacteria can show up and stay for a good long while.

So, do you have to give up flying? Stay home and watch travel videos instead? Not necessarily.

- Disinfect the immediate area around you with wipes or hand sanitizer. For the tray table, give it a wipe-down, or put a few drops of hand sanitizer on it, and use a tissue to wipe it around. Do this for the window shade and the armrests, too.

- Keep your hands well washed, and make sure to do so before handling food, after reading the magazine, adjusting the air vent, and any other activities that bring you into contact with surfaces inside the plane.

- Use your overhead vent to create a gentle breeze. This will circulate the air better, and keep viruses from settling in your area, if they're tempted to do so.

- Use a nasal spray beforehand and throughout the flight to keep your nose hydrated. Make sure it is just a saline solution with water, not one with medicine. It will keep your nasal passages from getting dried out in the cabin air, and the salt might help to kill or prevent germs from taking hold in your nose.

- Wear layers of clothing, so that only the outside layer comes into contact with plane surfaces. This layer can be washed when you reach your destination.

- If you're sick, try to cancel or rearrange your flight plans. Yes, this is not always possible, but it's a courtesy to others and may prevent you from getting sicker. If you must travel, wash your hands frequently, and wear a mask.

YOUR OFFICE
or WORKPLACE

The bad news: your office is fairly teeming with bacteria and potential viruses. But you probably already guessed that. Here are some sobering thoughts.

- Door handles, elevator buttons, work computers, desks and desk tops, meeting room tables, office telephones, copy machines, the watercooler, the restroom, the break room, the coffee machine, the microwave, the break room sink . . . all of them and more are likely covered in everyone's germs.

- These germs include everything from harmless bacteria to E. coli, campylobacter, salmonella, norovirus, flu, and a host of other nasties have been found in tests of typical office spaces.

- One study found over 25,000 organisms on a typical office phone!

- Microbes are also all over your keyboard, and anything else that you are touching frequently.

- The closed environment of many offices doesn't allow for a lot of fresh air to circulate, so germs can travel freely about the office. This can be especially bad during cold and flu season.

So, do you quit your job? Tempting as that may be, it's probably not necessary, sorry to say!

- Practice good hygiene, always. Wash your hands frequently, clean up after yourself if you eat at your desk, and keep a supply of hand sanitizer at all times.

- Keep some disinfectant wipes with you to rub down door handles on restrooms, handles on the fridge and microwave, etc. Encourage your colleagues to do the same. Leave some wipes in the break room and encourage your coworkers to use them.

- The potential for contamination in food areas is high. Keep the refrigerator clean. Set up a plan to rotate who cleans it, at least once a week, and make sure that everyone pitches in to help. Throw out old food and be careful about letting food items contribute to spoiling others near them.

- If you have shared workspaces and computers, clean off your computer keyboard regularly with a bit of a disinfectant rubdown. This will benefit everyone using it.

- Bring your own coffee mug or other drink container and take it home with you to wash. This is especially true if the break room doesn't have a dishwasher.

- See if working from home a day or two per week is an option. Especially since the advent of COVID-19, more and more workplaces have become accepting of the idea of letting employees do at least some of their work at home.

Try talking to your colleagues and boss about your concerns and see if you can get a group cleaning effort started that shares the work around to everyone. Make schedules and stick to them.

PUBLIC SWIMMING POOLS *and* HOT TUBS

Swimming pools, whether public or private, are a treasure of summer for many. Nothing feels as good on a hot day as a splash in the water. And since most pools have chlorine in them, they're safe and sanitary, right? Right? Well . . .

- Some surveys have shown that as many as one in five people pee in the pool when they think no one is looking. That's both children and adults.

- A CDC report showed that every year, about one in eight public pools, hot tubs, etc., have to be shut down, at least temporarily, for health violation reasons. One of the main reasons? Contaminated water. The main source of that contamination? Feces and diarrhea.

- Some dangerous bacteria, such as cryptosporidium, can live in chlorinated water for days.

- A stronger-smelling pool actually means that there is not enough chlorine in it.

- The red eyes you get from swimming don't come from the chlorine, but more likely from a mixture of urine, sweat, and other things floating in the water. Lovely.

So is the pool off limits from now on? Do you just have to sit in your bathtub (which carries its own risks)? Not necessarily.

- Don't go to a pool if you have diarrhea or any other intestinal complaints. Be courteous to other swimmers.

- Make sure that any young children who are not yet toilet-trained are wearing fitted swim diapers.

- Always shower before you go to a pool. Once again, a lot of the germs come from people getting into the pool without washing themselves. This is a good way not to contribute to that problem.

- If you're concerned about the chlorine content of a pool, you can buy tests trips to check it. The CDC recommends that public pools have a free chlorine concentration of at least 1 ppm. If it's less than this, it may not be a good idea to go for a swim.

- Try to swim with your mouth shut, to keep out as much water as possible. When you're finished swimming, dry out your ears.

- Wash your hands after a swim. Take a shower if you can. The more you can wash off, the better.

- Listen to make sure the pool pump is working properly.

Swimming pools don't need to be off-limits if you take a few precautions. However, if you or family members have compromised immune systems, using a public pool is probably not a good idea.

GYMS *and* SPORTS FACILITIES

10

People go to gyms to get healthy and fit, and it can either be inspiring or intimidating to see so many people working out and trying to improve themselves. But while fitness is a worthwhile goal, most gyms are filled with germs of all kinds and you could be picking up any number of them every time you go.

- Staphylococcus and MRSA can easily live in the sweaty, steamy environment of a gym.

- Studies have shown that over half of gym-goers complain about seeing other gym users not wash their hands after using the bathroom, meaning that they're taking their dirty hands right back out to all that shared equipment.

- Thirty to 40 percent of gym-goers confess to not wiping down their equipment (weights, machines, etc.) after using it. They just pack up and go.

- Gym showers can be coated in athlete's foot fungus, plantar warts, herpes simplex, and other awful things.

The gym doesn't have to be a horror show, if you take a few extra precautions.

- Wash your hands frequently throughout your workout.

- Consider wearing washable workout gloves if you don't mind wearing them. These can be removed and washed easily when you get home.

- Be wary of the showers. They can be crawling with bacteria, yeast, mold, and everything else you can imagine. If at all possible, take your shower at home.

- Bring disinfectant wipes or a spray to sanitize equipment before using it. You have no idea who was there before, or if the equipment has been cleaned properly in recent days. Try to touch handles on machines (stair-climbers, bikes, etc.) as little as possible.

- Don't go to the gym if you have a cold. You're only going to spread it around. Be considerate of others.

- If you have any cuts or breaks in your skin, make sure they are properly bandaged before using common equipment. Open wounds can provide an ideal entry point for bacteria.

- Bring your own towel. Don't use one provided by the gym, because you have no way of knowing how well it was washed or how it's been stored.

- Use a vinyl or plastic gym bag and be sure to give it a good rubdown with disinfectant before and after using the gym.

Most people would still say that the benefits of a good workout outweigh the minimal risks of contracting anything really nasty at your local gym. Just be sure to take extra care with a few of these concerns, and you should be fine.

While COVID-19 forced the closure of many movie theaters across the United States, they've always been places where germs also gathered to be entertained.

- Studies have shown the usual skin bacteria are present on movie theater seats, but they have also found higher than normal amounts of fecal bacteria, presumably brought in by people who didn't wash their hands in the restrooms. If you're touching the armrests, and then digging in to your popcorn or other snacks, you're putting that bacteria right into your mouth!

- Other studies have found streptococcus and even bedbugs lurking in the confines of cushy seats!

- Cupholders are, as you've probably guessed, teeming with bacteria. And these are rarely cleaned.

- When the staff cleans theaters, they're usually just picking up the big messes in between showings: popcorn spills, wrappers, etc. If a floor is especially sticky, they might give it a quick mop. But the seats? Not during the day! Seats may get an end-of-day vacuuming or maybe it'll be done once a week, but that's not going to remove the bacteria.

- Concession stands are supposed to be held to the same safety standards as any food service place, but let's be honest, they rarely are. Drink spills are common, and bacteria can thrive in them. One study found that 17 percent of disposable cup lids contained fecal bacteria. And how long has that popcorn really been sitting in the glass container?

So are movies a no-go from now on? Is it on-demand at home streaming for all of us? Here are a few suggestions for making movie theaters safer.

- Use some disinfecting wipes on the armrests, the cupholders, etc. Or wipe them with a bit of hand sanitizer and a napkin. It tends to be dark in theaters even before a movie, so you can get away with this without looking too weird!

- Wear long-sleeved shirts and long pants to a movie. Take them off and wash them when you get home.

- Don't place your coat on the floor, which is crawling with germs. Keep it in your lap. The same goes for purses and bags. Yes, that means you'll have to keep more in your lap as you watch the movie.

- Wash your hands before entering and after leaving a theater. Since there may be people in there sneezing or coughing, also try not to touch your face until you can wash your hands again.

- Leave your cell phone in your bag or pocket. Anything you touch is going to transfer to your hands and then right on to your phone screen.

- Monitor the cleanliness of the snack bar and buy (or not) accordingly.

More and more, people prefer to stay at home to watch films, but if you're a movie addict, there are ways to make the experience safer.

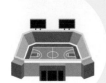

CONCERT HALLS, SPORTING EVENTS, *and* OTHER PUBLIC VENUES

The thrill of a good live show, whether a rock concert, an opera, a ballet, a musical, or a good piece of theater, is something we've all enjoyed at one time or another. And attending sports events is a tradition for many. But when you get a large number of people together, invariably, you're going to be bringing all kinds of bacteria and viruses to the show, as well.

- Seats are cleaned only irregularly. When you sit down in one to enjoy your show, there's no way of knowing what the last person (or the last twenty) have left behind that might be waiting to latch on to you.

- The floors may not be as dirty as a movie theater (fewer concert venues allow food inside, for example). But this just means that may be deep cleaned even less often.

- Rock shows in clubs are often standing-only venues, which is good for not picking up things from seats, but you're still surrounded by people inhaling and exhaling, probably more so than at a classical concert. There will be a lot more potential for viruses getting shared.

- Outdoor sporting events carry somewhat less risk, but when you get that many people together, it's inevitable that at least some are going to get sick.

But you don't necessarily have to give up on your love of live shows and events. Here are some simple actions to take to protect yourself. Many of these are the same as the recommendations for movie theaters.

- Use some disinfectant on the armrests, either wipes or a bit of hand sanitizer and a paper napkin.

- Don't leave your coat or bag on the floor. Set them in your lap.

- Keep your cell phone use to a minimum before the show, or don't bring it out at all. Anything you touch in the theater is going to get on your hands and go right to your phone screen.

- Take all the normal precautions you would in the restrooms, at the food counters, etc. All the extra people make these even more into germ hot spots.

- If you're sick, just stay home and be disappointed. Don't risk others' health.

Live performances of all kinds can be thrilling and a great way to bond with fellow fans. But it's essential to look out for each other, as well as oneself.

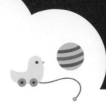

DAY CARE CENTERS, GYM CHILDCARE, *and* SCHOOLS

Anywhere that groups of children congregate is not going to be the cleanest environment! Head colds and other afflictions run rampant, and getting sick from one thing or another is basically inevitable.

- Obviously, being around other children puts all of them at an elevated risk not only for colds and flu, but all ear infections, diarrheal diseases, conjunctivitis (pink eye), pinworm, and other infections.

- Places with children will be crawling with bacteria. The general lack of handwashing among children and their tendency to get their fingers into everything will only make this worse!

- The younger the child, the more likely they are to get sick. It's estimated that children in kindergarten can get colds as often as twelve times a year, while by the time they are teenagers, this number drops to between two and four.

- For children who attend schools with cafeterias, bad news: germs are all over the tables and trays, and potentially in the food.

- Water fountains are a bit of a disaster. Kids often just put their mouth right over them instead of drinking from the stream.

- In all, a child may encounter over 150,000 germs in a day at school.

So how best to keep your child, yourself, and the whole family safe, or safer?

- Childcare institutions and schools have sets of guidelines for health and safety that they must follow by law. Investigate these and make sure that your place of choice is abiding by them. These include regulations about food preparation, immunization (for both children and staff), cleaning and sanitizing toys and other items, policies about children being sent home or staying at home when sick, and so on. These policies are usually posted and available to you.

- Make sure your child's immunizations are up to date and complete. Your pediatrician will have further guidance, and may recommend an annual flu shot, as well.

- Get your children in the habit of washing their hands properly and regularly. You can't control what other children do, but you do have say over your own child's actions and can explain the importance of keeping their hands clean.

- Keep your children's nails short and well-trimmed, as this will reduce the risk of bacteria getting lodged underneath them, and prevent other unpleasant things, such as pinworm eggs, from getting stuck there.

- Get your children in the habit of using their own water bottles, rather than relying on water fountains. Show them how to fill them, and make sure you wash them daily.

- Offer to donate disinfecting materials.

- Keep your children home at the first sign of illness. Help prevent the spread of anything further by isolating them.

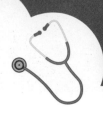

A DOCTOR'S OFFICE

We go to see doctors to improve our health. Unfortunately, a visit to the doctor's office runs the genuine risk of making us sicker, if we're not careful!

- Door handles in and out of the office, as well as inside the office itself, are potentially swarming with bacteria and viruses. They'll be cleaned at night (presumably), but during the day? Not a chance.

- Clipboards with forms almost always come with pens, and they're crawling with germs. In fact, studies have shown them to be one of the dirtiest items in the entire office!

- Armrests on waiting-room chairs? What do you think?

- Most offices have credit card machines, and these are just as germy as the ones at your local stores and ATMs.

Here are some ways you can reduce your risk.

- Wash your hands. It's always the best advice, and just as true here. Keep some hand sanitizer with you as well, for a quick rubdown after your appointment.

- Get your annual flu shot. This will reduce one major risk of being around others in an enclosed space.

- On that note, don't schedule your annual physical exam in the winter months, if possible. Go when colds and flu are less common. Obviously, if you have something that needs to be seen, you can't wait until a better time of year, but don't make unnecessary visits.

- Try to make your appointments for early in the morning. Fewer people have been in yet, and the office was probably cleaned overnight. That means fewer germs all around.

- Wear a mask. Even without the considerations of COVID-19, a face protection can be a smart idea.

- Don't read the magazines in the office; bring your own reading material from home. Who knows how many people have touched them over the months and years?

- If you're bringing your children, say to a pediatrician's office, bring their own toys or books from home. Don't let them handle anything in the office.

- Use your own pen when signing documents, not the one provided.

- If an office is especially crowded, you might want to consider waiting in the hall, until it's your time to see your doctor.

Visiting a doctor is important to maintaining your health but is not without its own risks. Be sure you take any necessary precautions, especially if you are immune-compromised or have other concerns.

THE HOSPITAL

If doctor's offices are bad, hospitals take it to a whole new level. Everyone who goes in for whatever reason can be at higher risk from the various viruses, bacteria, and assorted unpleasant things that are milling about.

- The numbers of antibiotic-resistant strains of bacteria are on the rise in hospitals. Patients run a greater risk of contracting these, and they are much more difficult to treat.

- One study from 2015 showed that, in the United States alone, about 687,000 hospitalized patients acquired Health Care Associated Infections (HCAIs). The numbers have only grown since then.

- Stethoscopes can have all kinds of germs, and while most aren't harmful, some studies have shown that traces of more dangerous germs can linger and transfer to the skin of a patient. Fortunately, they are regularly cleaned, but this is not a guarantee of safety.

- Doctor's white coats can also be covered in germs. Believe it or not, many doctors don't wash these as often as they should (daily), and they can quickly become a breeding ground for all sorts of things, including MRSA and gram-negative germs (such as E. coli). These coats can inadvertently come into contact with other patients, with items in the room, etc., and if not cleaned regularly, those germs accumulate and multiply.

What to do to keep yourself safe in the place where you're trying to get well? Many of the same general guidelines for a doctor's office apply here, if you are visiting, or have a short appointment. The point is to minimize contact with the objects in the hospital itself.

- If you are a patient staying for a day or longer, it's fine to express your concerns to staff. Ask that your room be cleaned daily (it probably will be), and for staff to wash their hands, especially if you have any extra health concerns. It's OK to ask them to wash again before examining you, changing bandages, etc.

- If you have concerns about a white coat, ask your doctor about it, and ask him or her to remove it.

- Ask your doctor if he or she would be willing to clean the stethoscope before using it on you, as a precaution.

- If you are staying overnight, try to get a private room. Being on your own in a hospital room has been shown to significantly reduce rates of accidental infections.

- If you are having an operation or procedure that uses invasive tools or items that will touch you, it's OK to ask how they are cleaned.

- You might be tested for antibiotic-resistant bacteria at some point. This doesn't mean that you have any infections; it is screening done as a precaution and is a good thing.

CHAPTER 5

MISCELLANEOUS GERMS EVERYWHERE

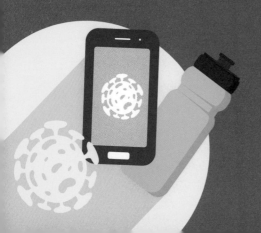

As we've seen, germs are pretty much everywhere, but we're not quite done yet! One of the most obvious places that you're probably aware of, but don't like to think about is your phone, and bad news: it's pretty gross! But what about paper money (yes, people still use it!)? Reusable water bottles? They're environmentally sound, but they can be magnets for all kinds of microbes!

And if you have pets, this opens a whole new (pet) door of germs into your life that you'll need to pay extra attention to if you want to keep your home as germ-free as possible. So delve into this final chapter to learn about even more places where germs are lurking to undo all of your hard work at keeping things clean!

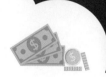

MONEY *(Bills and Coins)*

When you hear the phrase "dirty money," your mind may immediately jump to drug deals or an assassin's salary, but maybe you should take a more literal approach to this phrase. Why? Because studies show that fibrous US dollars may be one of the dirtiest objects in the world. It gives the phrase "laundered money" a whole new meaning! Here are some disturbing points to consider:

- The lengthy circulation of paper money (it can be out in the world for anywhere between eighteen months and fifteen years), multiplied by the number of people each bill comes in to contact with (imagine how many folks have handled that twenty in your wallet, and what they may have been up to!) creates a recipe for germ disaster.

- Just remember what a big deal washing your hands became after COVID-19; we started getting the impression that a lot of people really weren't doing it all that often or well before. Ew.

- Also, smaller bills see more action than larger ones; not too many people are flashing around Benjamins these days, but singles, fives, tens, and twenties still get a lot of use, so they'll typically have more germs.

Thankfully, the "cure" for this concern is already here, though it's come about for other reasons:

- With the nation's move towards automation comes a growing preference for cash-free lifestyles that favor credit cards and digital money apps over physical bills.

- No paper money, no problems!

- You may always need a little cash for certain things, but as we've gone more and more paperless and coinless (especially during the time of a scary virus), this is a problem that's pretty much taking care of itself.

- Still, if you do have to handle money, be sure to give your hands a good wash as soon as you can afterward. If you have to handle money for a living (such as at a bank), consider wearing lightweight cotton gloves while you do so.

Money has always had a germ problem, so the less often you have to use it, the better. But in some cases, traditional money is essential, so just be sure to keep your hands clean after handling it.

PHONES *and* PHONE CASES

We all love our phones. They're positively addictive. And you know what else is addicted to phones? Bacteria, viruses, germs, and just about everything else you can think of.

- One recent study found that there were more than 17,000 bacterial gene copies on the phones of typical high school students.

- Another study showed that phones can carry over 25,000 bacteria per square inch. This is far more than most doorknobs or even toilet seats.

- Indeed, a University of Arizona study revealed that cell phones generally have ten times more bacteria than most toilet seats. Think about that as you put it up to your face to make a call.

- Much of this bacteria is, as to be expected, neutral or harmless to humans. But this doesn't preclude the good chance of picking something less inviting, especially when you are out in public, handling your phone without have had a chance to wash your hands. And we all do that, all the time. MRSA, streptococcus, and E. coli. Have all been found on phone surfaces.

- In cold and flu season, the chances of picking up viruses on your phone go up.

- It's said that the average American now checks their phone eighty (!) times day. Just imagine how many germs that can spread around . . . .

So what to do? How do you keep your beloved phone at hand and stay healthy?

- Wash your hands frequently throughout the day, to keep down the spread of germs from your fingers to your phone.

- Try not to have your phone out with you in the toilet, especially a public one. The flushing will scatter bacteria around, and your unwashed hands will help in the spread.

- Clean the surface regularly with a microfiber cloth, like the kind used to clean eyeglasses.

- Disinfect your phone regularly with wipes, but make sure they are phone-safe; some are, some are not. Some phone companies make products or kits specially for phone cleaning.

- Some phones are waterproof, and you can spray them with a water and rubbing alcohol solution to disinfect. Be sure to check if it's OK to do this with your phone!

- Consider a UV light sanitizer if you use your phone out in the world heavily. These are a little pricier but can do a good job of killing bacteria on your phones glass surface.

- Don't use liquid sprays, which can harm your phone, unless they are specially formulated to clean phones and tablets. Spray on the cleaning cloth, never directly on the phone surface itself.

REUSABLE
WATER BOTTLES

These bottles have become all the rage. They're convenient, the metal ones can often hold hot or cold drinks, they're way more environmentally friendly than using plastic disposable bottles, and they're generally sturdy and can last a good long time. They're great for gym workouts, long cycling trips, keeping in your car, and any occasion when you need a quick drink of water without wanting to buy it in plastic bottles. But that convenience and even environmental consciousness might come at a price: your health and safety.

- According to one study, if you drink from a typical refillable bottle that you're not washing regularly, it's up to a hundred times worse than licking one of your pet's chew toys. Just chew on that for a minute!

- There could be a few hundred thousand colony-forming units of bacteria per square inch on your water bottle, all of which you're lifting up to your mouth every time you take a drink.

- Unwashed water bottles can be many times germier than pet food bowls or even your kitchen sink. Yuck!

- Another study showed that up to 99 percent of the bacteria on squeeze-top and screw-top bottles was of the gram-negative rods kind; this is the bad kind that you don't want anywhere near you! And up to half of the bacteria on slide-top bottles has been found to be harmful.

So, how do you put this portable germ factory out of business?

- Wash your bottle every day. If it's dishwasher-safe, put it in there with your nightly dish load and give it a good washing. If you wash by hand, hot water and a good liquid detergent will do the trick. Just be sure to rinse it thoroughly.

- It's probably not necessary to further disinfect it, unless you haven't washed it in a long time and film or slime is building up in places you can't see. Check the inside and the grooves and crevices to see if any reside is in them.

- Studies have shown that straw-top bottles seem to be the safest in terms of the least amount of harmful bacteria found on their surfaces.

- Metal bottles are a better and safer option than plastic ones.

You don't have to give up your more ecologically conscious bottle during your fitness routine. Just make sure you keep it as clean as possible, every day, and you'll drastically reduce the crazy amount of bacteria that can build up on it so quickly!

YOUR SHOES

Shoes are essential for going anywhere in the outside world; remember the old "no short, no shoes, no service"? Some people even turn them into an obsession (Imelda Marcos), or make funny videos about the craze ("Let's get some shoes!"). There's actually a lot to be said for going barefoot more often (it's good for overall foot health), but that's not an option most of the time. And because it's not an option, shoes are little more than germ buses and taxis. Pretty much everything you step on you can pick up in the outside world, and these get brought right back to your home: dirt, feces, urine, chewing gum, food particles, germs, bacteria, viruses.

- One study discovered nine species of bacteria on the shoes of the people who took part. Over the span of two weeks, researchers found about 440,000 units of bacteria on a single pair of shoes. One pair. That pair could be yours. It probably is, and you probably don't want to think about it.

- Another study found fecal bacteria on 96 percent of the shoes tested. Whether picked up in public restrooms or not, it was still there.

- Among the many kinds of bacteria that studies have found lurking on the soles of your shoes: E. coli, klebsiella (causes pneumonia), and bacteria that cause meningitis.

- Other substances, like toxins, herbicides, and plain old dirt love to stick to your soles.

There's no doubt about it, your shoes are probably the dirtiest thing you will wear today. So, what to do?

- Never wear your outside shoes in your home. Ever. Always take them off at the door and have a dedicated place to store them, such as a rack or washable mat. If you have a whole section of a closet devoted to storing your shoes, you might well have to rethink that situation. Do you really need that many, and if so, can they be houses closer to the front door?

- At the same time, don't just leave shoes outside. This can allow even more germs and bacteria to attach themselves to them.

- Keep the area around where your shoes are stored extra clean (the floor, the shoe rack itself, etc.). This will prevent the spread of germs that have decided to drop off your soles and go for a little wander in their new home!

- Keep your shoes clean. Depending on what kind they are, you might even be able to toss some of them in the washing machine. Otherwise, take your shoes outside, and use soap and water to spot-clean; this is especially good for the soles. Many insoles are washable. Take them out and soak them in soap and water. Let them air-dry.

We need our shoes, but we can't let them bring risks into our home. Keeping them away from most of your home is the best strategy. Plus, keeping them as clean as you can will reduce the spread of all kinds of nasty things from the outside world into your abode.

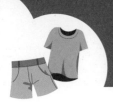

YOUR CLOTHING

Clothes make the person, but they also attract all sorts of invaders who'd just love to take up residence in their creases and folds. Everything that you brush by in the outside world can pick up something.

- Folding your coat over a chair or putting it on a floor, sitting in chairs, leaning against furniture or walls . . . all of it guarantees that you'll come into contact with strange and new bacteria.

- These visitors are brought back with you and are happy to jump off onto your sofa, your bed, wherever.

- If you are handling dirty laundry (putting it into the hamper, or taking it to the washing machine), you can easily pick up whatever germs are there and spread them all over your hands.

- When your clothes are in the washing machine, you may not be washing away germs. Instead, they can actually spread between various articles of clothing!

- Underwear will probably have more germs than outerwear, because of its proximity to your skin. Fecal bacteria, fungus, and other such things can easily find their way into these garments and jump on over to other clothing, if they sit in a hamper together for too long.

So, what to do about this seemingly unsolvable problem?

- Consider changing out of your clothes as soon as you get home, if possible. A lot of people can't wait to get out of their work clothes and into something more comfortable, anyway. So use comfort as an excuse to remove the day's garments and put them aside for washing. Keep them in a dedicated hamper; don't just throw them on the floor in the corner of a room.

• Wash your clothes regularly. Don't let them pile up for a week or more in the hamper (much less in a corner!), which will only give time for more bacteria to grow. This is even more important if you or someone in your home has been sick. The flu virus can survive for up to twelve hours on fabric.

• Use hot water when you can, though some items must be washed in cold water. Some machines have a "sanitize" cycle, which is good to use, if your clothing can stand it. It's basically an extra hot water rinse.

• Try to use a detergent with color-safe bleach, as this will help further to kill germs, and not just spread them around. Again, some clothing can't be bleached at all, so check the tags and be careful; you don't want to ruin your favorite garment!

• Dryers don't kill all germs, but they help. Dry is the enemy of the damp conditions that bacteria need to really grow. Alternately, it's great to hang clothes out in the sun to dry, as the sun's UV rays can do a number on those invasive little critters that are still hanging out in your favorite short or pair of trousers.

Taking a few extra precautions should ensure that your favorite clothes are not transmitters of things you'd rather not have anywhere near you.

YOUR FACE MASK

With the advent of COVID-19, people the world over have become accustomed to wearing face masks in public. The point of these, of course, is more to protect others from you, than to protect you from the outside world. But they do help serve both purposes, and they need to be kept as clean as possible in between trips outside. Of course, masks are worn for many other reasons: protection from smoke and allergens, by people undergoing cancer treatments and other medical procedures, and so on. In all of these cases, masks, like anything else, can get contaminated fairly easy.

Here are some important things to remember about mask cleanliness.

- Have more than one mask made of fabric that is washable. Two or three is ideal. That way, you're not stuck with the possibility of having to reuse your mask, should you need to go out again unexpectedly.

- If you are out, but away from others and want to take off your mask (say, in your car), remove it by the loops, and have some hand sanitizer ready to use after touching it. Try not to touch the front of the mask.

- Have a dedicated place, such as a bag, to put your mask in when you get home. Never just throw it on the couch or a side table.

- If your mask has filters, remove them and throw them away after each use.

- If you wear your mask until you get home, wash your hands thoroughly after removing it. Don't touch it again until it's time to wash it.

- Cloth masks can be washed in your regular laundry or soaked in a bowl of hot water and dish detergent, and then hand-washed.

- Or you can soak your mask in a water and bleach solution for five minutes first, before rinsing with cool water and washing. Use a bleach that contains 5.25–8.25 percent sodium hypochlorite and add four teaspoons to one quart of water.

- Dry your mask in the dryer, or let hang to dry. If you can dry it in the sun, even better, as the sun's UV will further help kill any remaining germs.

Masks are a way of life for most people these days, so keeping yours clean is essential to maintaining good health and staying safe.

CAT LITTER BOXES

Cats are generally clean creatures. They groom themselves frequently and are good about doing their business in their dedicated litter box. The occasional mishap notwithstanding, they can be counted on not to be too messy. Except when they can't! But in all cases, their litter boxes must be kept clean, because these contraptions, while good at keeping poop and pee in one place, can harbor some pretty nasty visitors if they're not cleaned regularly.

- A number of unpleasant bacteria and other creatures can be ingested by cats and excreted in their poop. These don't usually harm the animal, but they can be present in their excretions and transfer to humans. These include the bacteria campylobacter, the parasite Giardia (which can cause animal diarrhea), roundworms, and the parasite toxoplasma, which can cause all kinds of unpleasant symptoms in human and affect brain function.

- Outdoor cats are far more likely to have these infectious agents than indoor ones, since many of these infections come from eating raw or diseased meat, such as mice, rats, birds, etc. A cat that lives on canned wet food and packaged dry food will not be ingesting anything it shouldn't be.

The simple solution, of course, is to keep your litter box as clean as possible.

- Scoop out the litter box every day, even if there isn't much poop or pee in it. Some bacteria take a few days to become infectious after the feces are excreted, so if you remove it quickly, it won't have a chance to grow and potentially contaminate anything around it. Also, this prevents the buildup of ammonia from cat pee. While usually not dangerous to humans, the fumes can sometimes affect both cats and humans and cause headaches.

- Wash out the box weekly with hot, soapy water. Wear gloves and give it a good scrub, preferably outside. Clean the poop scoop as well, and only use it for this task.

- Pregnant women should not clean litter boxes. If toxoplasma is present and transmits to the mother, it can seriously damage the fetus.

- Have more than one litter box, if you have multiple cats.

- If you have a dog, be sure that it stays away from the litter box, so as not to pick up or transmit litter, poop, or infections around the house.

- Consider keeping your cat indoors. If this is just not possible, you'll have to take extra care when cleaning, and do it more often.

- Always wash your hands thoroughly after cleaning the litter box.

Fortunately, the risk of infection or contamination is fairly low. Taking a few extra precautions should be more than enough to ensure your safety and keep your kitty happy!

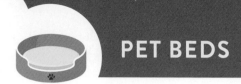

PET BEDS

Many of us like to spoil our canine and feline friend with their own dedicated beds. These are great for them, offering a familiar and comforting place to go whenever they want to. After all, we've all had days where we just want to go back to bed and stay there! But of course, pet beds can get dirty quickly, from hair dirt, and anything they may have brought in from outside.

- If your pet spends time outdoors, they're tracking in whatever they've come into contact with. Once they settle down on their favorite bed, those things can jump off and make themselves at home.

- Ringworm, salmonella, listeria, fleas, and MRSA have all been found in studies of pet beds, along with other yeasts and fungi, and random bacteria. Any of these can easily spread from your pet to its bed and then to other places in your home.

Fortunately, washing the pet bed can greatly reduce germs and dirt, and contribute to everyone's health, yours and your pet's.

- Wash your pet's bed regularly, at least once every two weeks, or preferably once a week. If they are exclusively indoor pets, you may be able to go longer between washes.

- Be careful, pet hair can ruin your washing machine! Hair clumps when it gets wet, and can cause clogs and real damage. If the pet bed has a removable, washable cover, always vacuum it first, or use a roller to get as much hair off of it as possible before putting it in the machine. If you get a lot of pet hair on your clothes and other laundry in general, be sure to use a roller to remove it before washing.

- Dry the cover in your dryer, if it's permissible to do so.

- If the bed doesn't have a cover, you can still wash it. Vacuum it first and then soak in the bathtub or a large basin with warm, soapy water for at least fifteen minutes, periodically pressing down on the bed to push out any trapped dirt.

- Drain the water and use a damp scrub brush to spread baking soda all over the bed. This will help to remove any lingering odors. Be sure to rinse it completely to get any remaining soda off.

- Squeeze excess water out of the bed and let it dry, preferably in the sun, if possible. Be sure it is thoroughly dry before putting it back into your place. Your impatient pet may not understand, but it's necessary!

Take the time to clean your pet's bed, just as you wash your own sheets and bedding regularly, and you'll keep their favorite sleeping place much cleaner and healthier.

PET TOYS

Dogs and cats love their toys. There's nothing more exciting than pawing at them, taking them in their mouths, chewing them, slobbering on them, and leaving a twisted spit-covered mess when they're done! Great fun for them, but then you're the one on cleanup duty.

- Toys that are in pet's mouths can easily become breeding grounds for things like coliform bacteria (which includes staphylococcus bacteria), molds, yeast, viruses, etc. Whatever else they've licked before will have transferred its germs to their mouths and tongues, and then onto their toys.

- If they are getting these toys in their mouths, or rubbing their faces on them, everything else they rub or lick in the home has a good chance of picking up whatever they've been chewing, including your hands or face, your sofa, etc.

Keeping pet toys as clean as is reasonable (and let's face it, they're going to get dirty quickly and often!) is important for their health and yours.

- Toys that are plastic, rubber, or nylon can probably be washed by hand in hot soapy water. Some may even be cleanable in your dishwasher (and may have instructions that this is safe). Since these will be going back into their mouths again after they are clean (thus undoing all your hard work!), *never* disinfect them with bleach or anything else that could be toxic! Stick with soap and hot water, and rinse them off thoroughly. Your pet isn't going to want the taste of soap in its mouth!

- Cloth toys, like stuffed animals, can be surface cleaned or often tossed in the washing machine (again, check for instructions). A good, hot wash followed by a tumble in the dryer should be enough to remove dirt and most germs. For some toys, they may need to be surface cleaned. Again, check the instructions. Try to do this once every two weeks or so.

- Be prepared to get rid of toys that have been chewed and handled to the point of falling apart. No matter how much your pet loves them, they could become dangerous. Things like dangling parts, loose string or fiber, and missing pieces can all become choking hazards, so keep an eye on their toys for when they get too worn. A rubber toy might be chewed to the point of having sharp edges or small pieces that can break off easily. Your pet may not be happy with losing a prized toy, but their safety is more important! Buy them something new as a distraction.

Pet toys, like children's toys, require a bit of monitoring for safety, and some effort to keep clean, but it's worth it when they have something they love and you can let them keep it for as long as possible.

IN-OUT PET FLAPS

A cat flap or a place where a dog can wander in or out offers a lot of convenience. Not having to be ready to open the door every time your pet wants to go out go come in is a great time-saver and lets them come and go as they please. The problem is, of course, that you have no idea what they'll encounter (or roll in) outside, and as soon as they come in, they'll be dragging it back inside with them. And the pet flap or door can be the first place some visitors drop off.

- As an animal scrapes through a flap or past a door, it will shed fur and maybe even skin cells. In these can be all sorts of bacteria and other things brought in from the outside world, which are now finding home on your floor or carpet.

- The door or flap itself can be a great place for bacteria to take hold and multiply, especially the side facing the outside world. So even if your pet doesn't pick up anything while outside (unlikely), it could still rub against a nice bacteria-infested door and then bring those little bugs inside when it returns. These microorganisms might stay on their fur, or feel free to drop off elsewhere in your home at their leisure.

Clearly, keeping flaps and in-out doors clean is essential as a first line of defense against outside invaders.

- Wipe the flap down with disinfectant or a one-part water to one-part white vinegar mix, to kill germs and keep the door odor and bacteria free. But be sure that your pet doesn't use it until it's completely dry. You don't want them getting anything on their fur and then licking it off! Alternately, hand clean with some soap and water every couple of days.

- Keep the floor near the flap extra clean. Dust, vacuum, and mop with a bit of disinfectant. Again, keep your pet clear of the door until it's completely dry, just as you would when cleaning any floor area in your home.

- Consider cleaning the outside floor or ground around the flap, too, to reduce bacteria and germs that may have set up camp out there. Sweep it up, and used an occasional water and vinegar scrub on the ground/concrete to kill germs.

- Make sure that your pet's flea treatments (collar or liquid) are up to date. Fleas can easily hitch a ride and jump off at the flap or in your home.

Since the flap is a pet's window to the world, it's essential to keep it as clean as possible. They will invariably bring things back in, so, make sure their doorway is as clean as you can keep it.

DOG LEASHES *and* OTHER PET SUPPLIES

Leashes, food bowls, blankets, and other such accessories are essential for an animal's well-being and happiness. But as you can imagine, they get germed-up pretty quickly, and you're going to have to make the effort to keep them clean more often than you might think. Here is a rundown of some of the more common things you'll need to clean and how to do it.

- **Food bowls:** Wash after every meal, if you can. You don't want them to become encrusted with old food, saliva, and germs, and your pet will appreciate having a fine dining experience! Plus, food and water bowls can quickly build up what is known as bacterial biofilm, a slimy substance that is covered in bacteria of all kinds, many of which can be dangerous. In addition to the obvious dangers to humans, these bacteria can cause any number of health problems in animals, including periodontal disease, inflammation, cardiovascular problems, and kidney infections. Most bowls can be hand-washed with soap and water or put in the dishwasher for a deeper clean. Check the instructions and see which one works best. It's a good idea to have more than one set of bowls and be sure to replace them if they become cracked, chipped, or damaged in any way.

- **Pet blankets:** These are much like pet beds and will get covered in fur and germs pretty quickly. Most often, you can just throw them in the washing machine. Consider washing blankets, bed coverings, and toys all in one separate load, if possible. Just remember to remove extra hair with a vacuum or roller first, so you don't screw up your washing machine!

- **Leashes and harnesses:** These are made of many different kinds of fabrics, leather, or other substances, and since they are worn around the neck or body, they will come into contact with whatever the pet is carrying on its skin. Some may be machine washable, and if so, you should wash after every use, just as you would your own clothing. Others may need to be hand cleaned. Check for cleaning instructions.

- **Animal carriers:** This is more for cats when being transported, but if you need to visit a vet regularly, you'll want to keep your carrier as clean as you can. Some are made of hard plastic and can easily be scrubbed out, while fabric and soft-shell ones are a little trickier to clean. Check if there are instructions for cleaning these, since you probably can't just toss them in the washing machine. Some topical cleaning with a damp cloth and baking soda may suffice.

Whatever accessories your pets have, it's important to keep them just as clean as anything else in your home, for their health and yours.

GARBAGE BINS *and* TRASH DISPOSAL

Garbage bins are for garbage (no kidding). That means that they are one of the dirtiest, germiest things you can come into contact with. Whether in your kitchen, other rooms in your home, or the outdoor ones that you leave for trash collectors, you're going to be tossing stuff in them constantly, and probably touching them regularly enough, and that means they'll need to be cleaned.

- The usual suspects, E. coli, salmonella, and listeria, all thrive in garbage can environments.

- Other substances, like mold, can easily take hold and start to grow in the dark, damp environments that a trash can offers.

- Larger creatures like maggots can easily spawn and take up residence in places with decaying meat and other food.

- Outdoor trash cans can attract flies, ants, and other insects, if food is left in them for too long, not to mention even larger creatures such as rats and wild animals.

Trash cans, both indoor and outdoor, need some extra attention given that they're germ magnets. Here are some tips.

- Use plastic bin liners or trash bags, or both. This will cut down on the number of germs that thrive in the bins themselves.

- Both indoor and outdoor bins should be cleaned regularly. Put on some rubber gloves, get the soap and hot water, a scrubbing brush, and sponge, and go for it!

- Soap and water may not be enough to get everything clean, to eliminate odors, or to properly disinfect a bin, though, especially if you haven't cleaned it in a while (which, let's face it, is most of us!).

- Add a half to three-quarters cup of chlorine bleach to a gallon of warm water and pour it into the bin or can. You can put the lid on and swish it around a bit, if you wish, though be careful about spilling. Let it sit for a least fifteen minutes, or longer if the bin is particularly dirty, and then, wearing gloves, scrub with a long scrub brush to get any remaining dirt and grime off the insides, and rinse thoroughly.

- Use disinfectant wipes or a spray to do a quick surface clean of the outside tops of bins, handles, etc.

- Clean your bins regularly, once every two weeks or more often, depending on how dirty they get. Consider renting a power washer if they get too gross!

Face it, you're never going to get rid of all the germs in a trash can, and as soon as you clean them out, the process will just start all over again! The trick is to try to stay ahead of it, at least a little.

A BRIEF LIST OF SOME HARMFUL BACTERIA

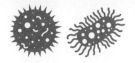

Here are some of the more common and dangerous bacteria, and what they can do (just in case you want to be even more worried!).

Acinetobacter baumannii: One of the highest-risk bacteria out there, it is, like many other types of bacteria, relatively harmless to healthy people, but for those who are compromised or injured, it can be deadly, attacking the blood, lungs, and wounds. The bacteria can cause pneumonia, meningitis, and UTIs.

Campylobacter: A cause of food poisoning, often found in raw or undercooked poultry, as well as contaminated water or milk. Symptoms are generally mild, but an infection can become deadly in children, older adults, and those with compromised immune systems.

Clostridium difficile (C. difficile): A type of bacteria increasingly common in hospitals, it can cause diarrhea and potentially damage the colon. C. difficile is treatable with antibiotics; the problem is that infections can come about because someone has already used antibiotics to treat something else, and this bacteria can take advantage of a weakened system.

Coliform bacteria: These bacteria are found in the feces of most animals. While they are less likely to cause illnesses themselves, if they are present in drinking water, it could indicate that other disease-causing pathogens are present. They are an indicator of drinking water quality.

Escherichia coli (E. coli): Most strains of this bacteria are harmless and can reside in our guts without doing anything, but there are a few varieties that can be quite dangerous. We hear about E. coli outbreaks pretty commonly these days, and they can cause food poisoning and even meningitis if left untreated.

Klebsiella pneumoniae: This bacteria has become more and more drug-resistant, and while generally not a danger to healthy individuals, it can cause, as the name suggests, pneumonia in immunocompromised people. It is often found in hospitals and other medical facilities, and can be spread by hand-to-hand contact, or on surfaces such as ventilators or catheters.

Listeria monocytogenes: This bacteria is often found in contaminated food, especially deli meats, and other lunch meats, such as hot dogs. Symptoms of infection are usually mild, but it can become much more dangerous for pregnant women and those over sixty-five. It can cause blood sepsis and swelling in the brain.

Mycobacterium tuberculosis: One of the great scourges of the nineteenth century, tuberculosis is making a comeback in the modern world in drug-resistant form. Between 10 and 13 percent of all new cases are now drug-resistant.

Neisseria gonorrhea: This dreaded STD is increasingly resistant to antibiotics, and cases that can't be treated are becoming more and more prevalent.

Pseudomonas aeruginosa: The World Health Organization classifies this form of bacteria as one of the greatest modern threats to human health. It's a nightmare bug that can be drug-resistant, and especially dangerous to people staying for longer times in a hospital, as it can reside on medical equipment that hasn't been cleaned well enough. It can cause pneumonia, blood infections, and UTIs, among other things.

Salmonella: A common source of food poisoning, drug-resistant strains have been found to be on the rise in Africa and Asia. It is commonly found in contaminated water and food, and in addition to food poisoning, it can cause a form of typhoid fever.

Staphylococcus aureus: The staph infection is well known and is usually a minor skin complaint. But if it gets into a wound, for example, and finds its way into your system, it can become deadly, affecting the blood, the lungs, the heart, even the bones.

Streptococcus pyogene: The infamous strep throat bacteria is a scourge that can lead to more serious conditions, such as scarlet fever. Up to 15 percent of all people carry these bacteria with no harm whatsoever, and even though it is still easily treatable with penicillin, versions with at least some antibiotic-resistant properties are becoming more common, causing worry among health care professionals.

ESSENTIAL CLEANING TOOLS

Here is a list of the most important items you need to keep your home and everything else in the best and cleanest state possible.

cleaning sponges: You'll want to have several on hand, each one with a designated job. *Never* use the same sponge that you clean dishes with to mop up spills or clean the counter. Always make sure that they dry out completely between uses, and replace them frequently.

disinfectant wipes: Various companies make these in different sizes. They are disposable and are great for cleaning things like handles on stoves, doorknobs, refrigerator handles, and so on. Keep a good supply handy so that you can run them over any areas, as needed.

dusters: Buy the kind with individual dusters and an attachable handle (such as Swiffer). These are design to grab hold of dust and trap it. A regular feather duster just scatters the dust around.

dustpan and broom: This set is always useful for something, such as a broken glass (though always vacuum, too, to get every bit of it), spilled dry food (rice, coffee, etc.), pet fur, dirt, and so on.

floor mop: There are many varieties of these, including several with disposable pads and containers that squirt cleaning liquid. Even a basic string mop is great to use after vacuuming to get out any ground-in dirt in kitchens, bathrooms, and from hardwood floors.

microfiber cloths: These are great for cleaning surfaces without leaving debris behind or scratches. Buy several at a time and you can wash and reuse them.

paper towels: Sometimes the most hygienic way of cleaning up a stain is with a paper towel, rather than a cloth one. You probably already have a supply on hand in your kitchen. Use them for cleaning and even drying as needed.

plastic buckets: Buckets are great for mixing water with bleach or vinegar, and it's good to have several different sizes on hand for different purposes.

plastic spray bottles: These are great for water-vinegar mixes and other solutions. They let you spray right where you need to clean. Just be sure not to let your mixture sit in the bottle for days or weeks at a time after cleaning!

rubber gloves: Protecting your hands when you get into grimy and dirty areas is essential. Have more than one pair and use them for different tasks for all of your cleaning, especially when cleaning drains, toilets, etc. Wash them by hand in soap and hot water after using and allow them to hang and drip dry.

scrub brush: You may want to have more than one, i.e., one for the bathtub, one of the sink, etc. These are great for getting deeper cleans.

soda crystals: Another nontoxic, all-purpose cleaner, soda crystals are great for using in washing machines, but are also good for clogged drains, grease buildups, and even cleaning tarnished silver. They are dissolved in warm water and then do their magic!

squeegee: This is a great tool for keeping your shower clean. Using it after a shower will help remove water and keep mold and mildew form building up. They're also great for cleaning windows, of course!

toilet brush and holder: You almost certainly have one of these. Be prepared to change it out a few times a year.

toothbrush: No, don't just use your old ones! Buy some toothbrushes and keep them just for cleaning small areas. They're great for tiles and for getting into small spaces.

vacuum: This goes almost without saying, but this machine is essential to keeping your floors clean. A **carpet sweeper** can also be useful for times in between vacuuming, when you want to freshen up the floors a bit.

white cloth towels: Sometimes you might need a cloth towel, so keep a supply of cheap cleaning towels on hand. Buy them in white so that they can be bleached easily.

ESSENTIAL CLEANING ITEMS

There are many products and chemicals which you can use for cleaning, from mild to harsh. You can buy commercial cleaners or make your own that are often just as effective. Here is a brief list of some of the more common liquids, powders, and soaps at your disposal.

all-purpose cleaner: The are a number of good all-purpose cleaners, including Simple Green, Microban 24 Hour, Mr. Clean Multi-Purpose Cleaner, Simple Pleasures Multi Surface Cleaner, Seventh Generation All Purpose Cleaner, and many more. You'll need to decide what your needs are, and the kind of cleaner you want to use, from traditional to environmentally friendly, or somewhere in between.

ammonia: This compound of compound of nitrogen and hydrogen has many uses in various industries. Ammonium hydroxide is a solution of ammonia in water, and is commonly used in cleaning. Ammonia has many cleaning uses, from ovens to bathtubs, to removing stains from clothing, to even reviving crystal glasses and getting rid of tarnish from brass.

baking soda: Like vinegar, baking soda seems to have hundreds of uses, from a cleaner to a deodorizer. Open a small box and leave in your refrigerator to absorb odors. Combined with water into a paste and spread onto surface, it cleans and brightens. It can unclog a drain and bring old stuffed toy back to life. Truly, it's a miracle cleaner!

bleach: Bleach kills bacteria and germs quickly and is an essential component of your cleaning cabinet. A mixture of one part bleach to nine or ten parts water is usually the right ratio to get things truly disinfected. Use care, since it is toxic and caustic. For safety tips, see the next section.

dish soap: Almost any kind of dish soap doubles as a good multipurpose cleaner, but it's especially helpful to get one that's formulated to cut through grease and oils, since this will work not only on food grease, but other kinds of oil as well.

glass cleaner: Windex and similar cleaners are great for getting your glass clean and streak free. You can also spray on a mixture of one part white vinegar to one part water, and wipe down your windows with newspaper, which will prevent streaking.

hydrogen peroxide: Another great nontoxic, all-purpose cleaner, hydrogen peroxide has multiple uses, everything from disinfecting your toothbrushes to cleaning kitchen surfaces. It kills germs and a tablespoon mixed into a cup of water can even revive plants and help reduce pests.

other scouring powders: Comet, Barman's friend, and other scouring powders have similar properties to baking soda and are useful for cleaning enamel and porcelain surfaces, such as sinks and bathtubs.

toilet bowl cleaner: Using a variety with bleach is a great option, and make sure that it is the kind that will stick to the sides of the bowl, as this will loosen up trapped dirt and make it easier to remove with your toilet brush.

white vinegar: A miracle, all-purpose cleaner, distilled white vinegar is great for cleaning most things. A simple one-to-one combination with warm water is great for so many different needs.

HOUSEHOLD CLEANERS THAT SHOULD NEVER MIX

While having so-called natural or old-fashioned cleaners on hand is useful and desirable, not all of them are meant to go together. Here is a list of combination no-nos.

bleach and ammonia: The combination can release vapors that will burn your throat and potentially cause respiratory damage. It can even kill you!

bleach and rubbing alcohol: Combining these two makes chloroform; you might end up knocking yourself out, and in higher doses, it can be extremely dangerous!

bleach and vinegar: The vinegar's acid will release toxic chlorine vapors that can cause chemical burns to the eyes and lungs.

bleach and pretty much everything else: If you haven't guessed yet, bleach should really only be combined with water!

hydrogen peroxide and vinegar: Combining these two produces paracetic acid, which can be corrosive to metal (such as taps and handles).

various household chemical cleaners: On their own, they may work perfectly well, but given the guidelines listed here, you need to be very careful about combining them, even if you check the ingredients of each. It's far better to use each cleaner independently.

vinegar and baking soda: These two are actually safe to mix, but only in certain circumstances. Remember those school science project volcanoes? Yeah, it will bubble up and go everywhere. This can be good for cleaning drains but use with caution in other areas.

vinegar and water for wood: The acid in the vinegar can damage the finish of floors and other wood surfaces, while the water will damage the wood over time. It's a great combo for cleaning other things, but for your floor, get a dedicated wood floor cleaner.

ABOUT THE AUTHOR

Tim Rayborn has written more than thirty books and dozens of magazine articles about various topics, especially on subjects such as music, the arts, history, business, and self-help; he will no doubt write more. He lived in England for many years and studied at the University of Leeds.

He's also a classical and world musician who plays dozens of unusual instruments from all over the world that most people of have never heard of and usually can't pronounce.

He has appeared on more than forty recordings, and his musical wanderings and tours have taken him across the United States, all over Europe, to Canada and Australia, and to such romantic locations as Marrakech, Istanbul, Renaissance chateaux, medieval churches, and high school gymnasiums.

He currently lives in Northern California with many books, recordings, and instruments, and a sometimes-demanding cat. He tries to keep things clean, but understands that the battle with cat hair will never be won. He's quite enthusiastic about cooking excellent food, though less enthusiastic about the cleanup afterward.

www.timrayborn.com

INDEX

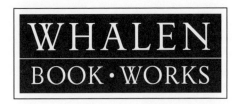

PUBLISHING PRACTICAL & CREATIVE NONFICTION

Whalen Book Works is a small, independent book publishing company based in Kennebunkport, Maine, that combines top-notch design, unique formats, and fresh content to create truly innovative gift books.

Our unconventional approach to bookmaking is a close-knit, creative, and collaborative process among authors, artists, designers, editors, and booksellers. We publish a small, carefully curated list each season, and we take the time to make each book exactly what it needs to be.

We believe in giving back. That's why we plant one tree for every ten books we sell. Your purchase supports a tree in the Rocky Mountain National Park.

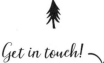

Get in touch!

Visit us at **Whalenbooks.com**
or write to us at
68 North Street, Kennebunkport, ME 04046.

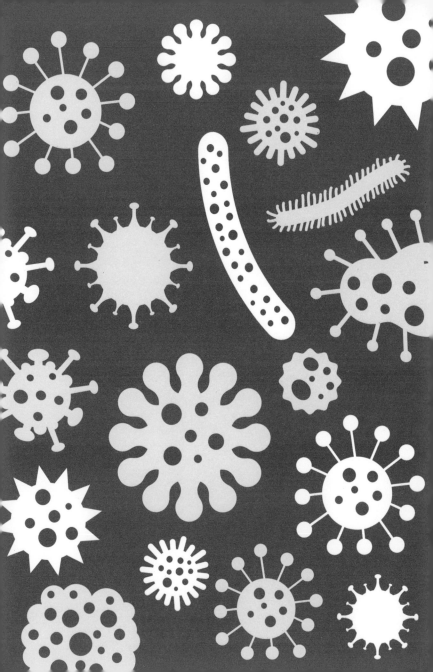

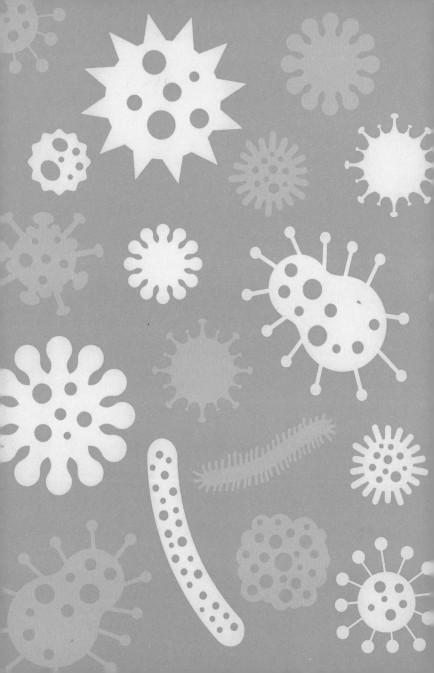